As Miss Nightingale Said . . .

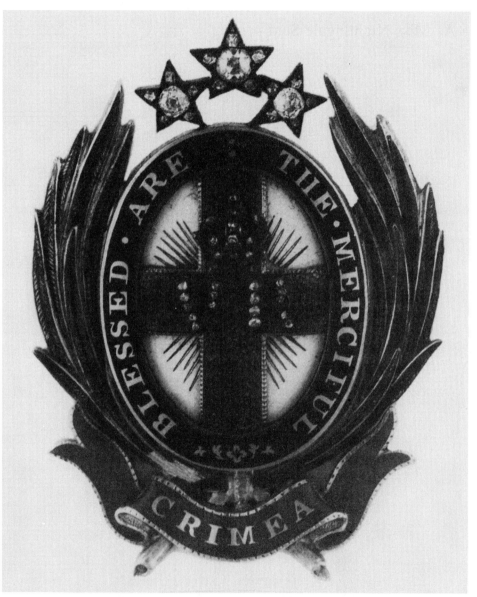

Brooch designed by Prince Albert and given to Miss Nightingale by Queen
Victoria during the Crimean War (photograph courtesy of the Director, National
Army Museum, London)

As Miss Nightingale Said . . .

Florence Nightingale Through Her Sayings –
A Victorian Perspective
2nd edition

Edited by

Monica Baly
FRCN SRN SCM HV PhD

*Researcher for the Nightingale Fund Council;
formerly Regional Officer, Royal College of
Nursing, London, and Lecturer and Examiner
for the Diploma in Nursing*

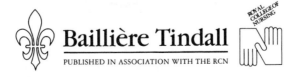

Baillière Tindall
PUBLISHED IN ASSOCIATION WITH THE RCN

London • Philadelphia • Toronto •
Sydney • Tokyo

Ballière Tindall   24–28 Oval Road
London NW1 7DX

The Curtis Center
Independence Square West
Philadelphia, PA 19106–3399, USA

Harcourt Brace & Company
55 Horner Avenue
Toronto, Ontario, M8Z 4X6, Canada

Harcourt Brace & Company, Australia
30–52 Smidmore Street
Marrickville
NSW 2204, Australia

Harcourt Brace & Company, Japan
Ichibancho Central Building
22–1 Ichibancho
Chiyoda-ku, Tokyo 102, Japan

A catalogue record for this book is available from the British Library

ISBN 0-7020-2292-6

Typeset by Keystroke, Jacaranda Lodge, Wolverhampton
Printed and bound in Great Britain by Hartnolls Ltd, Bodmin, Cornwall

In memory of Trevor Clay
whose wise leadership has
been an inspiration to nurses

Contents

List of Illustrations

List of Illustrations

Foreword

It is only in the last decade that Florence Nightingale's true place in history has come to be appreciated and acknowledged. Much has been learnt from the scholarship of Monica Baly, the author and compiler of this fascinating book of quotations, and Joyce Prince. The fact that the Nightingale nurse training school at St Thomas's Hospital, in which she took little interest at first, failed to fulfil the hopes invested in it, does not diminish the important role which she played in the history of nineteenth century social policy. The acknowledgement of her whole life's work is now fairly represented in the museum dedicated to her in the grounds of the hospital where her best known endeavour proved so difficult to realise.

It is a paradox that she should be best known for what she failed to achieve – a credible training for nurses in the school to which her name was given. This story is at last well documented. The St Thomas's school gave no more than a menial apprenticeship with very little instruction let alone education. It was run by an increasingly muddled martinet and such education as there was, was given by a doctor who was often inebriated and whose morals were questionable. The design had been laid down but never properly implemented. It was years before she came to know the truth. And when she did she made sure that the public did not. Glowing accounts continued to be written for public consumption. If the truth had come out, the success she had had in popularising nursing as a suitable and safe occupation for educated women would have been seriously jeopardised. And when she did know, the attempts at reform were by faint-hearted patch work. Everything might have been different if she herself had played a much more active role in the creation and supervision of the school from the start. But by this time she had (for whatever reason) adopted the role of a lifetime invalid and her interests had widened far beyond that of nursing.

As is well known, Miss Nightingale built her public reputation on her work in the Crimea. This established her in the public mind as 'an authority'. This and the social connections established through her family enabled her to establish herself as a one woman pressure group for social reform, operating largely behind the scenes. But her experience in the Crimea seems also to have given her an appreciation of the essential goodness of the soldier or 'the common man' if given education, opportunity and a sanitary home environment. And the most important opportunity was that of work. Thus she had the courage to dismiss the conventional wisdom of the day that work was always available for those willing to do it and that those who would not work had to be punished in the forbidding institution of the workhouse. Thus in her view the whole system of the Poor Law was rotten to the core. It did not just need piece-meal reform or rigid inspection but total redesign. Her solution, though not worked out at great depth, had remarkable similarities to that proposed much later by the Webbs in The Minority Report on the Poor Law of 1909.

She had the ear of those who mattered. Eminent men in a variety of fields were prepared to work hard and with little recognition for her pressure group. She had no need of headed writing paper or the cover of an Association. She had no need to lead deputations or agitations. All she needed to do was to write letters and memoranda from her couch in South Street and summon to her those whose brains she needed to pick or whose support she wanted to enlist. She was the first woman to have achieved in her own right a position so eminent and so wide ranging in the causes for which she fought. At different periods of her life she was fighting to reform the administration of the army and particularly its medical services, to change the system of hospital design and hospital location, to transform the emphasis of colonial policy in India from economic exploitation through railways to economic development through irrigation, to develop public financed hospitals for the poor and to extend preventive medicine from sanitation to what we would now call changing the lifestyle of the poorer classes through health visitors and community nurses. Her foresight was amazing. And all this is reflected in these quotations from her extensive private letters and published writing.

Like many of us she lacked consistency. She did not always practise what she preached. She was ambivalent in her relations with her family. She changed some opinions during her life and clung to others, long after her position could no longer be sustained in the light of the evidence. She was not always right. But she had a remarkable ability to see through to the core of a question. She realised that giving women the vote was far from being enough to give them equal rights to the extent that she saw this as a desirable aim. While she may have been misguided in her attitude to the registration of nurses, she was right in seeing that the status of nurses depended much more on what they were recognised as being able to do for society than on any formal legal protection of the occupation. Her vision of the role of the nurse extended beyond skills in applying techniques or procedures to seeing the promotion of health in all its aspects in lifestyle as well as environment.

She herself was respected not just because of the public image which had been built around her but because she had worked hard to acquire a wide variety of skills. She built on the man's education which her father had given her. She learnt to be an administrator and a manager and understood how organisations really worked. She became expert in the infant study of epidemiology. She understood about architecture, drainage and sanitation. And she had learnt how to write persuasive memoranda built upon hard evidence and use language with polemic effect.

This book of quotations brings this remarkable woman to life. It shows what she stood for and what she stood against. It demonstrates the breadth of her interests and yet shows the complex self-questioning of her inner life. She stands revealed, warts and all.

Brian Abel-Smith

Acknowledgements

Many of the quotations in this book originated in research undertaken on behalf of the Nightingale Fund Council, which resulted in *Florence Nightingale and the Nursing Legacy*, and I acknowledge the help of the Council, particularly to the late Sir Desmond and to Lady Bonham Carter and my supervisor, Dr W. D. Bynum, at the Wellcome Institute. My research meant long hours in the British Library and the Greater London Record Office, and I am grateful for the help received from the staff, especially Mrs Howlett at the Greater London Record Office. My thanks are also due to the Earl of Pembroke for allowing me to see the relevant papers at Wilton House, to Sir Ralph Verney and the curator at Claydon House, and for the help given by Mrs Sutton at the Wellcome Institute.

I should also like to record my debt to Susan McGann, the archivist at the Royal College of Nursing, for allowing me access to precious editions of Miss Nightingale's writing and for her encouragement and support.

My thanks are also due for the wise criticism and helpful suggestions of Professor June Clark, to whom I owe the inspiration of the title, whose sitting room floor was strewn with cuttings, scissors and paste as we reassembled the quotations.

Finally, my thanks go to Patrick West, the Editor of Scutari Press, who has been a counsellor and friend of nurse authors for many years, and to Trevor Clay who showed great interest.

In preparing the second edition of this book I am grateful to Anne Bassett, lately of Scutari Press, who encouraged the undertaking and helped with the first edition. I am also grateful to the Royal College of Nursing Library in finding, and allowing me to borrow, Florence Nightingale's works on religion, which are complex, long and often obscure. In comprehending them and reducing them to a few pages I am grateful to Prebendary Richard Askew, Rector of Bath Abbey, for his interest in 'this fascinating – and maddening lady' and to the Reverend Dora Frost, both of whom have endeavoured to guide my erring theological footsteps. My thanks are also due to Baillière Tindall who inherited this book and agreed to publish it.

Sadly, since the publication of the first edition the dedicatee, Trevor Clay, has died, as has the writer of the Foreword, Brian Abel-Smith, both of whom are sadly missed. However, I am glad that I did manage to capture a little quintessential Abel-Smith when I did, and I am eternally grateful for his encouragement and support for my research and its publication.

Preface

When asked by Scutari Press to expand the first edition, we decided that a new chapter, 'On Religion', would be a useful addition. Firstly, because the subject was avoided before as being too difficult and not fitting into the scheme of a lighthearted book; secondly, because there has been a burst of interest in the subject, especially in the United States; thirdly, because Church men and women find her spiritual struggle amid the conflicts and doubts of the nineteenth century both fascinating and relevant. Undoubtedly spiritual motivation was a driving force behind much of Florence Nightingale's work. She saw it as God's will and God's law that we should teach ourselves and that 'mankind should help mankind', and her whole attitude to the social problems of the day and to health care depended on her interpretation of God's law.

Another aspect of Florence Nightingale's life to attract attention since the first edition is the nature of her illness and why she was confined to her bed, or her couch, for so long? Generally our interest in the health of the famous lies with those who accomplished much, often against ill health, and who died comparatively young. Mozart, Keats, Schubert, Shelley, the Brontës, D. H. Lawrence and that long list of nineteenth century consumptives immediately spring to mind. What might they have accomplished had they the benefit of modern therapy and lived longer? Florence Nightingale is different. She thought, as did everyone else, that she was going to die in 1857 (at the age of 37 years), but she lived to the age of 90 years. In history what people think is happening is often as important as what actually happened. Did the prospect of imminent death drive her to work ever harder to avenge what she saw, and rightly saw, as the unnecessary suffering of the Crimea? On the other hand, did the sequelae of her 'Crimean Fever' (probably brucellosis) cause restless agitation and an emotional state that, in itself, drove her on? Did one factor act on the other, and to what extent were they compounded by her treatment? Since 1988 I have met with at least ten different diagnoses offered by medical and nursing historians as to the basis of her illness. To Florence herself it was 'The Thorn in the Flesh'. How she worked out a *modus vivendi* to cope with the 'T in the F' is important because her isolation and peculiar lifestyle had its down side as well as its positive results. Cut off from the realities of life beyond that upper room in South Street she became out of date, she was seldom contradicted, except possibly by Jowett, and she never saw more than one person at a time. In her letters we occasionally get sad glimpses that she is aware of how artificial her life is, but, she maintains, this is the price it was necessary to pay 'for the sake of the work'. If at times she seems harsh and hectoring we must set that against what she did achieve. Great reforms are not made by just being pleasant.

Monica Baly
1996

Preface to First Edition

Miss Nightingale was a legend in her own day. From the time she returned from the Crimea she was seen by many and was presented in the media of the day – from pictures to popular ballads – as saint and heroine. The tradition persists: it is still common to find Miss Nightingale, or something that she said, quoted as the justification for all that is good or bad in modern nursing and health care.

Hagiography is bad history, and myths are, by definition, misleading. If we look at what Miss Nightingale actually said and wrote, we are better able to sift the wheat from the chaff, and can begin to see that the nursing legacy associated with her name was not what she intended.

This is not a eulogy but an attempt at a balanced picture of this often misunderstood, enigmatic, eminent Victorian. The quotations, which do not pretend to be comprehensive, have been chosen to illustrate Miss Nightingale's thoughts on a variety of topics. Some are chosen because they are pithy and axiomatic, some because they are relevant today, while some illustrate her patrician point of view and show her fallibility.

Although the quotations are in general grouped according to topic, they are also presented, as far as possible, in chronological order, reflecting the various phases of Miss Nightingale's long and sometimes contradictory life, and in an attempt to show the development of her thoughts. Although this chronological ordering is important, it is well to remember that Miss Nightingale was nothing if not inconsistent. Sometimes it is clear that her views have changed over time, sometimes there are contradictions and inconsistencies in her views on apparently related subjects.

Readers may wish to use this book in either of two ways. Those whose primary interest is Florence Nightingale herself will probably begin at the beginning and read on, using each chapter like a piece of jigsaw puzzle to build up a cohesive, though never comprehensive, portrait. For those readers, I have been careful to name the source of each quotation and to give, where necessary, a note of the context in which the words were spoken or written. Since the sources of many of the quotations are letters from Miss Nightingale to the various members of a large, extended family and an ever-growing circle of distinguished friends, I have included a 'Who's Who' and some genealogical tables, which show how complex her social and political network was.

Other readers, however, may simply want to dip into the kaleidoscope in search of a *bon mot* for a speech or a quotation to support a point of argument; these readers may find it more useful to start with the list of contents or the index, look up the subject about which Miss Nightingale 'must have said something', and follow the numbers to find what she 'really said'. One way is not better than the other; this book is written for both groups – indeed for anyone who has ever found themselves saying, on whatever occasion, 'As Miss Nightingale said . . . '

Monica Baly
1991

Introduction

'I have taken effectual means that all my papers shall be destroyed after my death.'

Private note, 25 January 1864 (British Library)

For over sixty years of her life Miss Nightingale was a prolific writer. In her youth, she wrote private notes on scraps of paper, recording her hopes, dreams and fears. All her life she was a tireless correspondent to a wide range of distinguished and interesting people. Because the Victorians had more space, and also because, after 1855, the writer was famous, the recipients kept her letters and eventually donated them to one of the collections. However, Miss Nightingale is exceptional in the quantity of her written material because of her isolated lifestyle after 1857. Much of her day-to-day communication was done by letter; she wrote what she would have said. For example, Dr Sutherland, her amanuensis and adviser on sanitary matters, worked in a room in her house in South Street and, partly because of his deafness, she communicated with him on scraps of paper with such missives as:

'What has become of the 8 copies of the Indian Report?'

'Where is Barbados?'

'What am I to say about this arsenic wallpaper?'

These notes, together with his often amusing replies, are held in the British Library. However, for Miss Nightingale's views on nursing and the Nightingale Schools, we are indebted to the hoarding instincts of Henry Bonham Carter, her lawyer cousin and Secretary to the Nightingale Fund Council from 1861 to 1914. Henry who, unlike his predecessor Arthur Clough, did not live on her doorstep in South Street, did most of his communication by letter, preserving Miss Nightingale's often long replies in his papers, now housed in the Greater London Record Office.

Apart from the wealth of private correspondence, there is Miss Nightingale's published output. In his *Life of Florence Nightingale*, Sir Edward Cook [1] lists 147 printed publications, and this does not include all her letters to *The Times* and those many nineteenth-century magazines to which she wrote. Then there are drafts housed in one place, while the fair copy is preserved elsewhere. No scholar can read it all, or would wish to, for 'Oh, eternity is all too short' and some of it is tedious or trivial. When Miss Nightingale scribbled notes to her friends and collaborators, she was using paper in the way we use the telephone, and few of us would like our telephone conversations to be recorded, especially our more slanderous asides. However, at times she was writing for a wider public; when, as she got older, she found writing more difficult, and Jowett and Stuart Mill helped with drafts, she complained that 'they tidied up my purple prose and took out my *bon mots*'. The *bon mots* were carefully thought out.

In evaluating Miss Nightingale's writings, it is important to set her in her contemporary context. As a young woman she was a radical. She was influenced by the liberal views of her family and, in 1848, when travelling in Europe during the revolutions, she wanted to go to the barricades. Her views on women's property rights and the right to paid occupation were, in the 1840s, definitely avant-garde. As she grew older, though, she grew more conservative, but, like the angry young men of a later era, in old age she still regarded herself as a radical. The one-time champion of women's emancipation refused to support women's suffrage, and the idea of women doctors was anathema to her. She clung like a limpet to the concept of 'miasma' as a cause of disease, though, to give her her due, she did modify her views in old age. There is a delightful letter in which she accuses the matron of St Thomas's, Miss Gordon, of being unable to accept new ideas on infection not long after she herself had crossed out 'milk for children should be boiled' in a textbook by Florence Lees. Miss Nightingale was nothing if not inconsistent. On the other hand, in her seventies, she showed remarkable prescience in sanitary matters and the need for health education. Her views on the Poor Law and its operation were, and remained, iconoclastic. Had she been active in 1904, she would have been a supporter of Beatrice Webb and the Poor Law Reform Group [2].

Another subject on which Florence Nightingale appears to be inconsistent is religion. When the Nightingale Fund was launched in 1855, it was thought that it would be used for training nurses based on a religious order. The unfortunate Sidney Herbert, the chairman of the Fund, met opposition from the press and the public on the grounds that Florence Nightingale supported Socinianism (a doctrine akin to Unitarianism). Other opposition said she lent to 'Romanism', while the Anglicans said she was 'Low' or 'Broad' Church. A letter had to be published in *The Times* pointing out that the Fund was not connected with any religious group.

The critics had a point. During her long life, Florence Nightingale, like so many Victorians, went through many vacillations in her attitude to religion. She was a child of her time. Her parents had been Unitarians; Fanny's family had been associated with Wilberforce and a number of liberal causes. W. E. N., her father, had stood as a Whig MP with distinctly radical views. The girls were brought up on the philosophies of the Enlightenment and Florence was a competent classical scholar, in later life able to help Benjamin Jowett with his translation of Plato's *Republic*. W. E. N., himself had been educated at Cambridge, but because dissenters were excluded from English universities until 1828, many friends and relations had been educated in Germany where they were exposed to the philosophies of Shopenhauer, Hegel and Engels and new Biblical criticism. Among the friends from Germany was Chevalier Bunsen, Ambassador to the Court of St James 1842–54, who made a great impression on the young Florence. Bunsen was a scholar of ancient and oriental languages who had introduced Max Müller to Oxford and whose *Sacred Books of the East* had caused controversy but who had given a new sense to non-Christian religions. It was through Bunsen and another family friend, Julius von Mohl, married to Mary Clarke, that Florence became interested in comparative religions. Another acolyte of the Bunsen circle was Monckton Milnes, who spent five years trying to persuade Florence to marry him. Apart from social reform and philanthrophy, German philosophy was something else they must have had in common. We assume that Florence knew nothing of his collection of pornographic material . . .

Meanwhile the Nightingale family had become, at least nominally, members of the Church of England. This was largely because, having inherited property, they assumed squirearchial and parochial duties which they took seriously. However, while she was interested in new scholarship and scientific discovery, Florence was a serious young woman given to introspection and always searching for a purpose in life. At the age of 17 years she received what she felt was a 'call from God', and this gave her an affinity with mystics like St Teresa of Avilia, John of the Cross and Thomas à Kempis, whose lives and works she studied avidly.

While she was in Rome in 1848, sympathising with the *Risorgimento*, she spent a period in the Convent of Trinita De Monti, receiving instruction from Madre Sta Columba on the steps she needed to take to submit herself to the will of God. It was an experience that had a profound effect, and she contemplated joining the Church of Rome. Later, in 1853, she wrote to Cardinal Manning, an old friend, sending him a copy of *Suggestions for Thought* (see Chapter 3) for advice on conversion. Not surprisingly, Manning said her views were too radical. Nevertheless, one of the greatest influences on her continued to be Mother Clare Moore (Mother Bermondsey) who remained a guide on spiritual and nursing matters until Mother Clare's death in 1874. All her life Florence Nightingale continued to feel that the Roman Catholic church had more to offer women than the Church of England, with which she became markedly out of sympathy and which was having one of its fissiparous episodes with the Tractarians and their heirs, the Anglo-Catholics, at odds with the Evangelicals and both at war with religious liberalism.

Florence Nightingale was not alone in her equivocal attitude to religion in trying to reconcile the new scientific and historical approach with the inherent need for faith. Some, like her cousin, Arthur Clough, who had a great influence on her, had lost their faith in the teachings of the Church and resigned their academic posts. Matthew Arnold, Clough's friend, and an author of biblical criticism wrote in *Dover Beach*:

'The Sea of Faith
Was once, too at the full, and round earth's shore

. . .

But now I only hear
Its melancholy, long withdrawing roar . . . '

Others contemplating the 'long withdrawing roar' were Robert Browning, Alfred Tennyson, Beatrice Potter (later Webb), George Eliot and Harriet Martineau, to mention but a few. Some went though the dark night of the soul and, like Tennyson, returned to faith; others, like George Eliot, remained agnostics.

The whole history of the Victorian Church is shot through with conflicts aroused in individuals as they came to terms with new knowledge, and after 1859, Darwin and *The Origin of Species*. It is not surprising that the thoughtful, earnest Florence Nightingale in the course of a long life should go through many vicissitudes. Like her views on nursing education, she can be quoted, usually out of context, to support any religious view.

Another era in which Florence Nightingale appears inconsistent is her literary style. As Lytton Strachey [3] put it:

> The author of *Notes on Nursing*, that classical compendium of the besetting sins of the sisterhood drawn up with the detailed acrimony, the vindictive relish of a Swift, now spent long hours composing sympathetic addresses to Probationers whom she petted and wept over in turn.

Today we find Miss Nightingale's more fulsome and sentimental letters to her friends, and particularly to her favourite nurses, such as 'dearest little sister', 'Goddess Baby' and 'Pearl', and her fussing over their health, cloying, but Miss Nightingale was a child of her time and the effusive style was fashionable, with the recipient replying in kind – 'adored chief' and so on. Every age has its own epistolary style.

When Miss Nightingale died in 1910, the main events of her life were already history, the Crimean War was a generation ago, and her official biographer, Sir Edward Cook [1] and her literary executor, Henry Bonham Carter, were of necessity selective in the material they used. Miss Nightingale herself had written: 'memoirs written so soon after death if true are offensive, if not they are twaddle' [4].

This memoir was a eulogy and written immediately after death. The rough places were made smooth and the failures swept under the carpet. There were reasons for the cautious approach – there were personal and legal considerations, some of the people involved were still alive, or, if not, relatives were watching; reputations were at stake. As far as nursing was concerned, there was the delicate question of the relationship of the Nightingale Fund with St Thomas's Hospital. More and more the Fund was becoming irrelevant to nurse training, and Henry Bonham Carter's relations with the treasurer were strained; it would not have helped to open up old wounds by relating the battle about the site of St Thomas's or the Nurses' Home, or the sad saga of Mrs Wardroper and Mr Whitfield. Moreover, although, by 1910, nursing was established as a profession, it was now facing competitors, and the inspiration of the legendary founding figure was good for recruitment.

Because Cook's two volumes were so monumental and well written, most other biographies have been a shadow of them. Subsequent historians have generally only done new research on one aspect. Mrs Woodham-Smith [5] admitted that she had done little work on the nursing schools. More than anyone else, nurse historians have perpetuated the myth. They have conveyed to generations of nurses that the

Nightingale School was independent, that St Thomas's was Miss Nightingale's first choice, that Mrs Wardroper was a 'woman after her own heart', that the probationers were carefully chosen and 'were neat, lady-like and above suspicion' and they 'trained to train', and that this unique revolution spread quickly round the world. Early nurse leaders, anxious to portray nursing as an educated, homogenous profession, to be publicised as such, tended to overstate the horrors of what they called 'the Sairey Gamp era' and exaggerated the Nightingale reforms. There was no dramatic break in 1860. The Nightingale School was a small experiment, and at first a not very successful one, among the reforms already begun and already inevitable.

It is important to remember this today as we discuss the merits of a new system of educating and training nurses. If we had looked at the reality of what Miss Nightingale actually said about the defects of the apprenticeship system of training at St Thomas's, a reform of nursing education might have come sooner.

In assessing Miss Nightingale's writings there are three main pitfalls: her love of exaggeration; the confusion of her public and propaganda statements with her private comments; and the sheer span of time – in sixty or so years, she changed her mind many times.

First, the hyperbole which she used in an inordinate manner to make her point: sometimes the dramatisation leads to the apophthegm, such as 'it is the first duty of the hospital to do the patient no harm'. Sometimes, however, her histrionics are intemperate and lead to the accusations that she was a liar, as made by Professor Barry Smith [6]. Henry Bonham Carter wrote, when Miss Nightingale was complaining that Mrs Wardroper was acting like 'a semi-insane king by divine right': 'you are strongly impressed with, and inclined to magnify the deficiencies of character and conduct you have known, and do not give them credit for all they may be entitled to.'

Miss Nightingale was always inclined to raise everything an octave. There was no suffering like her suffering, no grief like her grief, no burden of work like hers: 'I have little more to do in each day than can be done in 24 hours,' she wrote to William Rathbone when she was 54 years old and living in South Street with a staff of five. Of course, the exaggeration and drama paid off. Being at 'death's door' and 'life hanging by a thread' concentrated her friends' minds wonderfully. For example, she pushed through the contract with St Thomas's against the better judgement of her Council by using that tactic. Sidney Herbert, himself a sick man, wrote in November 1859: 'She is failing badly; it will be a relief to get this thing out of the way.' Miss Nightingale had just sent him her 'last letter'. When she looked like not getting her way she had palpitations, nausea or had not slept for seventeen nights. It worked. Such self-dramatisation would have been reprehensible had it not been for the fact that the cause was generally righteous and the end justified the means. We can forgive the piling of Pelion on Ossa if it resulted in the reform of the army medical services, the sanitation of India, the midwifery services or the Poor Law. We can forgive the inflated invective if it drew attention and brought forth improved nursing services in civil and military hospitals and, above all, in the homes of the poor.

The second pitfall, and the one into which most biographers, including Cook and Mrs Woodham-Smith, have fallen, is to confuse public rhetoric and propaganda with private opinion. Miss Nightingale and the prestigious Nightingale Council were past masters in the art of public relations. They wrote letters to *The Times*, articles in magazines and addressed public meetings extolling the success of the 'reformed' nursing at St Thomas's, while privately they bewailed the failure to find suitable candidates, and 'after ten years we have only produced two super-intendents', and 'the probationers are doing half the Hospital's work', and 'St Thomas's is the unmaking of us'. While publicly praising St Thomas's, they were writing about the officials in a manner that was positively libellous: the Resident Medical Officer was 'more often tipsy than sober', the treasurer was 'cunning and unscrupulous' and 'we are not dealing with gentlemen', the latter being a repeated cry. Indeed, one of the mysteries of the Nightingale papers is, why did not the cautious, legal-minded Henry Bonham Carter destroy some? Miss Nightingale sometimes indicated that such letters should be burned, but this seldom happened. Historians are of course glad that the papers survive because they shatter the myth that Miss Nightingale regarded the Nightingale School as a success, or that it produced those 'trained to train'.

The same applies to Miss Nightingale's assessment of people. If it would serve the cause, Miss Nightingale could turn her hand to the most graceful panegyric and obituary notice. The classic example is the character sketch of Mrs Wardroper, published after her death in 1892 in the *British Medical Journal* and quoted by every biographer:

> She never went a-pleasuring, seldom into society. Yet she was one of the wittiest people you could hear on a summer's day . . . She moved in one piece. She talked a great deal but never wasted herself in talking. She knew what she wanted and did it. She was a strict disciplinarian, very kind, often affectionate . . . [7]

From about 1867 to 1887, the archives are full of letters of bitter complaint about Mrs Wardroper's incompetence, the failure to know one probationer from another, the muddling of the accounts, the absurd insistence on making nurses stand to atten-tion when she came in, the tearful states and the incoherence. Such criticisms were not confined to letters to Henry Bonham Carter, but there are sarcastic references to Mrs Wardroper's mental state in letters to favourite probationers, some of whom were equally candid about 'our dear matron'. Bonham Carter wrote that he did not leave 'matters that required judgement' to Mrs Wardroper. He nevertheless wrote a warm, if slightly elliptical, tribute on her retirement.

Agnes Jones is another example. Miss Nightingale never wanted her at St Thomas's; she was afraid that her religious zeal would upset the hospital. In the end she could not refuse because she was the niece of Sir John Lawrence, her friend and the Governor of India. As the only educated candidate, Agnes was sent to Liverpool to reform the nursing in the Brownlow Poor Law Institution. Agnes was Irish and there were 'Hiberian rows', which Miss Nightingale and William Rathbone mollified. Then the overzealous and overworked Agnes caught typhus and died after long death-bed scenes and 'last words', which were transmitted to Miss Nightingale. On hearing accounts of Agnes and 'miracles', Miss Nightingale thought that 'due to lack of sleep in the last months Agnes's mind had begun to turn'. But Agnes died a martyr to the cause of nursing and martrys are good for publicity. Miss Nightingale seized her pen and wrote 'Una and the Lion' for *Good Words* [8]. This starts with a sentimental eulogy about 'Una' (Agnes), but the main article is a hard-hitting appeal for women to come forward and nurse; it was blatant advertising for the Nightingale School. However, 'Una' should not be taken as Miss Nightingale's personal view of Agnes, whom she considered to be 'more interested in her Bible work than in nursing'.

Another example of Miss Nightingale's dichotomy between public pronouncement and private feeling is in her attitude to the family. Publicly and in letters to Clarkey (Madame Mohl), she made great diatribes against the suffocating effect of marriage ('the most selfish of institutions') and the family; but in spite of adolescent battles, Miss Nightingale seems to have been devoted to her family, as her letters from Rome [9] and Egypt show. She constantly thanks her father for the excellent education he gave her, as well she might. Later, she uses her ever-generous mother, Fanny, to look after sick Nightingale nurses or send flowers and evergreens to the Nurses' Home. Interestingly, Professor Barry Smith [9] fulminates about the closeness of the Nightingale clan fostering the reputation of their most famous member, while Mrs Woodham-Smith [5] stresses the family conflict. It is all confusing. It is true that Miss Nightingale thought that Victorian families stifled their daughters, but that is not to say that there was not a strong bond of affection in the family.

The third pitfall is the sheer span of time. During fifty or so active years, Miss Nightingale changed her mind many times. Like the Reverend Chasuble's sermon on 'the manna in the wilderness', she can be adapted for any occasion. You can use her to support one portal of entry to nursing (Briggs or Project 2000) or a separate officer class (Horder). You can use her to claim that working-class girls without much education but with the right motivation make the best nurses, or, on the other hand, 'only the educated will rise to the post of superintendent'. She appears to support the idea of a powerful businessman as a hospital administrator (Griffiths) and is against democratic committees and consensus. However, in nursing matters, she maintains that the matron must be supreme. This she achieved, and it was one of the most important parts of the Nightingale package. It is always said that she made nursing a 'profession', but late in life, reading the proofs of a book by Amy Hughes, a Nightingale nurse, she crossed out 'profession' and put in 'vocation'. Thirty years earlier, she had said she wished 'to found a normal school for professional nurses'. Like many people since, she is using 'professional' in different senses.

Miss Nightingale's writings are full of contradictions, but they can be partly explained by the great changes in hospitals, in medicine and in women's education during a fifty-year span. In *Florence Nightingale and the Nursing Legacy* [10], I argued that, contrary to received wisdom, the time was *not* ripe for reform in 1860.

Twenty or so years later, medicine was more scientific and doctors were more ready to see the need for trained, educated and hygienic nurses. The middle classes were starting to use hospitals and expecting good nursing, while more girls were being educated and had expectations of earning a living in a respectable occupation. The better educated wanted something more than routine work, so they carved out a role on the medical model. For a comparatively short time, nursing offered a career with few competitors. Hospitals, anxious to meet the new demands, capitalised on the fact that nursing was fashionable. With plenty of candidates, trainee nurses were exploited. This was the missed opportunity. Miss Nightingale never intended that probationers should be the main workforce of the hospital, and this is why, one senses, in the end she was disillusioned with the way nursing was developing.

Nevertheless, dramatisation, hyperbole, contradiction and, dare we say it, sometimes with an elliptical regard for the truth notwithstanding, Miss Nightingale in some matters had a remarkable prescience and has left us with thoughts that are timeless, and, when her pen was dipped in gall rather than treacle, that are witty and worth remembering.

References

[1]   Cook Sir E (1913) *The Life of Florence Nightingale*. 2 vols, London: Macmillan.
[2]   Baly M E (1986) *Florence Nightingale and the Nursing Legacy*. London; Croom Helm (paperback edn 1988).
[3]   Strachey L (1918) *Eminent Victorians*. London: Chatto and Windus.
[4]   Nightingale F (1860) *Letter to Baroness Bunsen*.
[5]   Woodham-Smith C (1950) *Florence Nightingale*. London: Constable.
[6]   Smith F B (1982) *Florence Nightingale – Reputation and Power*. London and Canberra: Croom Helm.
[7]   Cook Sir E (1913) ibid., vol. 1, p. 458.
[8]   Nightingale F (1868) 'Una and the Lion', *Good Words*, June.
[9]   Keele M (ed.) *Letters from Rome Written by Florence Nightingale 1847–1848*. Pennsylvania: American Philosophical Society.
[10] Baly M E (1986) *Florence Nightingale and the Nursing Legacy*. Conclusions, p.219. London: Croom Helm (paperback edn 1988).

1

A Victorian Family

The nineteenth century saw a new phenomenon, that of well-to-do women becoming idle in the home. Until the industrial revolution, for most women the whole business of living had taken up most of the day. Now, with an ever-increasing number of labour-saving devices and a growing army of domestic servants, there was less and less for upper- and middle-class women to do. In many ways, the Nightingale family was typical; there were two houses in the country, Embley and Lea Hurst, and the season in London. In other ways, however, it was not typical; both parents were liberal in their outlook and Florence and her sister Parthe enjoyed an education that normally would have been bestowed on a son with a private tutor.

Miss Nightingale's early life should have been happy; the family travelled a great deal and entertained much, and there were dozens of close relatives, most of whom were interesting and intelligent. Mrs Nightingale always had a host of distinguished guests. Florence was intelligent and attractive, and she 'shone in society'; she obviously enjoyed her education with her father and was an apt pupil. Her private notes, however, have that tragic and dramatic tone that was to become characteristic of her. She was introspective and thought of herself as 'different'. When she was seventeen, she had a 'call' from God, but she was not sure what God wanted her to do. She became obsessed with the misery of the poor, and in 1844 she realised that her 'call' was to nurse, but she did not know how to nurse – she needed to be taught. This led to her plan to go to Salisbury Hospital – and a family row. The family have had a bad press, but their reluctance to let their accomplished daughter go into the squalor of a hospital is understandable, and there was plenty of other good work she could do. They hoped that Florence would marry, and they encouraged Monckton Milnes, for whom there is no doubt that Florence felt affection and admiration.

Monckton Milnes was an interesting man, a poet of distinction, a literary critic of discernment (he discovered Keats) and a philanthropist. As a Liberal MP he was not a persuasive speaker, but he continued to support Miss Nightingale's causes in the House. Later, as Lord Houghton, he was a trustee of the Nightingale Fund and a valued member of the Council until his death. When Florence went to the Crimea, he wrote: 'You could undertake the East when you could not undertake me.'

Parthe, Florence's sister, had more sense and talent than Mrs Woodham-Smith allows. She was active in working for the Nightingale Fund and she writes a good, sensible letter with her feet firmly on the ground and was loyal to her sister, though not impressed with her capacity as a nurse. She was a competent artist and later wrote five novels, and, when she married Sir Harry Verney, she helped him to run his estate.

One suspects that, with her dreaming and introspection, Florence was a rather difficult young woman, who must have appeared ungrateful. But we have only Florence's version of life at home. We do not know what the Corinthians thought of St Paul. Florence's main complaint, as voiced in her unpublished novel of 1852, *Cassandra* (which appears in Vol. 2 of *Suggestions for Thought*), was of the triviality of much of the household round and the lack of personal time for the unmarried woman to develop her own interests and work. She felt that God required her to do something more useful that just reading aloud to papa, entertaining company or visiting with mama.

'Dear Pop, let us love one another better than we have done. It is the will of God and Mamma particularly desires it.'

to Parthe, 1830

'Dearest I am looking forward to next Sunday, if I can be tacked on to some-body's apron string – how often I wish for grey hairs – they are the greatest possible convenience – and, if they could be had before other infirmities would be as much an advantage as Brevet Rank.'

to Hilary Bonham Carter, 3 May [?]
1840

'The morning is spent sitting round the table in the drawing room looking at prints, doing worsted work, reading little books. Everybody reads aloud from their own book or newspaper and every five minutes something is said. The afternoon is passed in taking little drives. . . . When night comes women suffer physically the accumulation of nervous energy which had nothing to do all day and makes them feel every night when they go to bed as if they are going mad.'

Suggestions for Thought, Vol. 2,
Cassandra

'What is my business in this world and what have I done this fortnight? I have read the *Daughter at Home* to Father and two chapters of Mackintosh, a volume of *Sybil* to Mama. Learnt seven tunes by heart. Written various letters. Ridden with Papa. Done company, that is all.'

Private note, July 1846

'I must have some leisure to find out a few things.'

Private note, 1841

'It must be for fun I try to make them understand me – because I know it is impossible.'

Private note, 1851

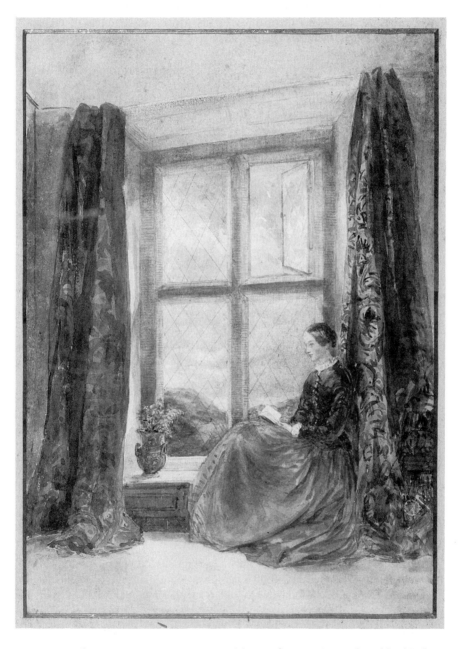

Florence Nightingale at Lea Hurst, painted by Parthenope (reproduced by kind permission of Sir Ralph Verney and the National Trust at Claydon House).

'The family uses people *not* for what they are, nor for what they are intended to be, but what it wants them for – for its own uses. It thinks of them not as God has made them, but as the something it has arranged that they shall be.'

Suggestions for Thought, Vol. 2,
Cassandra

'The prison that is called family, will its rules ever be relaxed, its doors ever opened? What is it, especially to the woman? The man may escape and does.

But what are we to do with the girls? It is vaguely taken for granted by women that it is to be their first object to please and obey their parents till they are married. But the times are totally changed since those patriarchial days. Man (and woman too) has a soul to unfold, a part to play in God's great world.'

Suggestions for Thought, Vol. 2

Further on in this chapter Florence Nightingale writes about the time when Christ was told that his mother and brothers were waiting. Instead of being angry he said:

'Who is my mother? and who are my bretheren? Whosoever shall do the will of my Father which is in heaven, the same is my brother and sister and mother.'

Florence Nightingale goes on to say:

'If we were to say that, we should be accused of "destroying the family tie" of "diminishing the obligation of home duties".'

Ibid.

'O God, no more love, no more marriage. Oh God.'

Private note, 1846

'Rubbed Mrs Spence for the second time. I am such a creeping worm that if I have anything of the kind to do I can do without marriage or intellectual or social intercourse. . . . It satisfies my soul. It supplies my every want of heart and mind . . . '

Private note, July 1846

'We must all take Sappho's leap one way or another before we attain her repose – though some take it to death and some again to marriage and some again to a new life even in this world. Which is the better part God only knows.'

to Mary Clarke on her marriage to
Julius Mohl, 1847

'I have an intellectual nature which requires satisfaction and that I would find in him. I have a passionate nature which requires satisfaction and that I would find in him. I have a moral and active nature that requires satisfaction and that I would find in his life. Sometimes I think I will satisfy my passional nature at all events, because it will at least secure me from the evil of dreaming. But would it? I could be satisfied to spend a life with him combining our different powers in some great object. I could not satisfy this nature by spending a life with him in making society and arranging domestic things.'

Private note, Summer 1849
(On refusing marriage with Monckton
Milnes.)

'I know since I refused him not one day has passed without my thinking of him, life is desolate without his sympathy.'

Private note, 1849

'Last night I saw him again – he would hardly speak – I was miserable.'

Private note, March 1851
(On seeing Monckton Milnes again.)

'Why, oh my God, can I not be satisfied with the life that satisfies so many people? I am told that the conversation of all these clever men ought to be enough for me. Why am I starving, desperate and diseased on it? . . . My God, what am I to do?'

Private note, 1851

'In my thirty first year I see nothing desirable but death.'

Private note, 1851

'The water-cure is a highly popular amusement within the last few years amongst athletic individuals who have felt the *tedium vitae* and have indefinite diseases which a large income and unbounded leisure are so well calculated to produce.'

Florence Nightingale's Note book,
quoted by Cook, Vol. 1, p. 118
(On accompanying her father to a spa in
1852. She herself was to take the waters
at Malvern in 1858 but was sceptical
about their value.)

'To avoid lying long in bed, and the temptations of the world, liking to be praised and admired and a general favourite more than anything else [to which] we were both very much affected.'

Private note, 1841
(Quoted Woodham-Smith (1950) p. 51.)
(Advice to her favourite nephew William
Shore, who was to inherit the
Nightingale property. He was 14 years
old and she 21.)

2

The Call

From the time she was seventeen, Miss Nightingale felt that she had been called by God for a special mission, but she was not sure what. Then in 1845, witnessing sickness among the rural poor, she realised that lives were lost for want of proper nursing and hygiene. Unlike her contemporaries, she was convinced that nursing required training. But where was she to find such training? The next eight years were spent in trying to find a preparation and reading those weighty nineteenth-century reports on health, social and sanitary matters known as the Blue Books. She visited hospitals on the continent and used her time abroad to look at nursing by religious orders.

During this period, she made two visits to the Protestant deaconesses at Kaiserswerth on the Rhine. The first was a brief visit of observation, but on the second occasion, she spent several weeks working with the deaconesses. Miss Nightingale denied that she was 'trained' at Kaiserswerth, since she thought they knew little about nursing, but she was impressed with the fine devotion to their charges from working-class girls. This influenced her when she was considering who would make the best nurses at the Nightingale School.

One of the difficulties with the Nightingale family life at this time was the fact that the two sisters, both gifted, seemed incompatible and at times got on each other's nerves to the distress of their parents. Although Parthe was devoted to her sister, she obviously envied her social success and she was fearful that Florence would indeed leave home. Mrs Woodham-Smith (1950) paints a picture of Parthe as being childish and hysterical, which does not seem to be borne out by Cook (1913, vol. 1), and, of course, we only have Florence's side of the story. If Parthe had a 'breakdown' in 1850–51, could it not be that she too was frustrated and thwarted and, like her sister, at the age of 30 years, was wondering what her fate was to be? Although not as intellectual as Florence, she was well educated, a gifted artist, vivacious, fond of literature, with a prose style more euphonious than that of her sister, and she was elegant (which Florence was not). When Florence was in the Crimea, Parthe gave sensible and practical advice about the Nightingale Fund. On becoming Lady Verney she ran the household, and helped with the estate and the archives with what seems commendable efficiency.

In her calmer moments, Florence admitted that Parthe had talents that she lacked and an appreciation of art and nature that she envied. Although the situation may have been difficult in 1849–51, Florence does seem to have dramatised it.

Apart from family opposition, there was the problem that there was little nurse training; she had to train herself as best she could by reading and observing. In August 1853, thanks to the influence of aristocratic friends, Miss Nightingale became the unsalaried Lady Superintendent of the Invalid Gentlewomen's Institution in Harley Street. The position was made possible by a generous allowance of £500 from her father. She took the appointment seriously and was her own work-study expert. This was the breakthrough; she could organise, and she came in touch with several eminent doctors who became her friends for life.

Although the private notes are full of lamentations about 'seeing nothing in life but death', during this period Miss Nightingale travelled, went to the opera, became 'music mad' and enjoyed society. One senses that there was a tension between the demands of human relations and society, and a desire to break out of the circle and do something 'to the glory of God'. It was God versus Mammon, and it was this conflict that accounted for her periods of depression and the conflicts with her family.

'On February 7th 1837 God spoke to me and called me to His Service.'

> *Private note, 7 February 1837*
> *(In 1874, Miss Nightingale recorded that*
> *God had spoken to her through her*
> *'voices' four times.)*

'In making myself worthy to be God's servant the first temptation to be overcome is the desire to shine in society.'

> *Private note, 1839*

'My mind is absorbed with the suffering of man, it besets me before and behind, a very one sided view but I can hardly see anything else and all that the poets sing of the glories of this world seems to me untrue. All the people I see are eaten up with care or poverty or disease.'

> *Private note, Summer 1842, Lea Hurst*

'I saw a poor woman die before my eyes this summer because there was nothing but fools to sit up with her, who had poisoned as much as if they had given her arsenic.'

> *to Hilary Bonham Carter, December*
> *1845*
> *(Hilary was a favourite cousin and the*
> *brother of Henry, q.v.)*

'You will laugh, my dear, at the whole plan [to be a hospital nurse], but no one but the mother knows how precious the infant idea becomes; nor how the soul dies: . . . I shall never do anything and am worse than dust and nothing . . . '

> *to Hilary Bonham Carter, December*
> *1845*

'This morning I felt as if my soul would pass away in tears, in utter loneliness, in a bitter passion of tears and agony of solitude. I cannot live, forgive me oh Lord, and let me die this day, let me die.'

Private note, 1845

'My life is more difficult than almost any other kind. My life is more suffering than any other kind, is it not God . . . ? Let me diminish the suffering of my life knowing that I *cannot* what I so truly desire, minister to Parthe's happiness while in such suffering myself God's Law has provided against that . . . '

Private note, [?] 1851

'To be cheerful and gentle with Parthe – that is my object. Now, how is it to be obtained? Not by violent effort, nor by pretence and falsehood, but by clear understanding of her character and mine and by the laws influencing such characters.'

Private note, June 1851

'I am blamed by everybody, most of all by themselves, "for seeking duty away from the sphere in which it has pleased God to place me" . . . It is only known that my sister has bad health & what can I be doing away from home nobody can understand . . .

I know you will pray for us . . . '

to the Reverend Henry Manning, 1852
(Manning had recently converted to
Rome.)

'I believe I shall go for the present to the duty nearest at hand – to nurse a sick aunt – and wait and see what I can find out to be God's work for me.'

ibid.

'Remember that you know what is the real object of life better than you did, better than many who have not suffered, and, if you like, ruined. Remember that you believe in God and will become one with him

to offer a religion to the working Tailors

to translate the prophets.

If you carry out these objects they will keep you healthy.

Why can't you get up in the morning? I have nothing I like so much as unconsciousness but I will try.'

Private note, [?] 1851
(Florence Nightingale started on
Suggestions for Thought to the Searchers
after Truth among the Artizans of
England in 1852 (see Chapter 3).

'Today I am 30 – the age at which Christ began his mission. Now no more childish things. No more love, no more marriage. Now Lord let me think only of Thy Will, Oh Lord Thy Will, Thy Will.'

Private note, 12 May 1849, Athens

'The nursing there was nil. The hygiene horrible. The hospital was certainly the worst part of Kaiserswerth. I took all the training that there was to be had – there was none to be had in England, but Kaiserswerth was far from having trained me. . . . the tone was excellent and admirable. And Pastor Fliedner's addresses the very best I have ever heard . . . his solemn and reverential teaching to us of the sad events of hospital life was what I have never heard in England.'

Recollections of Kaiserswerth, 1897

'I have never met with a higher tone, purer devotion than there. There was no neglect. It was the more remarkable because many of the Deaconesses had been only peasants – none were gentlewomen. The food was poor. No coffee but bean coffee. No luxury; but cleanliness.'

*Note in the British Library with the
pamphlet she wrote on the training at
Kaiserswerth, 1851, sent 1897*

'This is the life. Now I know what it is to live and love life, and I really would be sorry to leave life. . . . I wish for no other earth, no other world but this.'

*to Mrs Nightingale (Fanny), July 1851,
from Kaiserswerth on her second and
longer visit to the Institute*

'My Committee refused me to take *Catholic* patients – whereupon I wished them good morning unless I might take in Jews and Rabbis to attend them . . . from philanthropy and all the deceits of the Devil, Good Lord deliver us.'

to Mme Mohl, 20 August 1853

'To scour is a waste of power.'

*to the Committee, on installing labour-
saving devices at Harley Street*

'My dear I must have them boots. . . . More flowers, more game, more grapes . . . '

*to Mrs Nightingale, 1854
(Miss Nightingale's feet were hurting
and she was sending to 'dearest mum'
for boots made by her personal boot-
maker. 'Dearest mum', as usual, was
generous in supplying her daughter's
needs.)*

'I am now in the heyday of my power . . . '

to Mr Nightingale, 1854

'Our vocation is a difficult one . . . and though there are many consolations and very high ones, the disappointments are so numerous that we require all our faith and trust. But that is enough. I have never repented or looked back, not for one moment. And I begin the New Year with more true feeling of a Happy New Year than I ever had in my life.'

to her cousin Marrianne, now married to Douglas Galton (q.v.), later Lady Galton, January 1854

'I gained a very curious experience while there while managing the former class [hysterical governesses]. I had more than one lunatic. I think the deep feeling I have for the miserable position of educated women in England (or rather half educated) was gained there. But I would not undertake it again, I would begin nearer the source. Physicians were of little help to me, they rather made matters worse. For patients looked on medical attendance as a luxury.'

Recollections of Harley Street to Dr Pincoffs, a doctor friend from Scutari, written in 1857

'When I entered into "service" here I determined that happen what would I *never* would intrigue among my Committee. Now I perceive I do all my business by intrigue. I propose in private to A. B. or C. the resolution that I think A. B. or C. most capable of carrying in Committee, then I leave it to them and I always win.'

to Mr Nightingale (W.E.N.), 1853

'The nurse should never be obliged to quit her floor except for her own dinner and supper and her patients dinner and supper.

Without a system of this kind the nurse is converted into a pair of legs for running up and down stairs. She ought to have hot and cold water, she ought to sleep on her own floor in her own bedroom.'

to Lady Canning, Paris, June 1853
(The system of the Sister sleeping in a
room off the ward and taking the name
of the ward continued in some hospitals
until well into this century.)

'We have no funds to have an accountant and if we had he would be off with the money.'

to Mrs Nightingale, 1853
(Part of a long letter thanking the ever
generous Fanny for all her gifts to the
Harley Street Home.)

'The opinion of others concerning you depend not at all, or very little, upon what *you* are but what *they* are. Praise and blame alike are all indifferent to me. My popularity is too great to last.'

to Mr Nightingale, September 1853

'My Committee are such children in administration. . . . The place is exactly like administering the Poor Law. . . . My Committee have not the courage to discharge a single case. *They* say the Medical Men must do it. The Medical Men say *they* won't, although the cases they say *must* be discharged. And I *always* have to do it, as the stop gap on all occasions.'

to Mr Nightingale, 1854

'The chemists sent me a bottle labelled Spirits of Nitre which, if I had not smelt it, I should certainly have administered it and we should have had an enquiry into poisoning . . . '

to Mr Nightingale, 1854

3

On Religion

Sir Edward Cook described Florence Nightingale as 'a passionate statisician' [1]. She was, however, not only a passionate statistician but a passionate sanitarian who believed that statistical methods used by Jacques Quetelet could be applied to the problems of health. Quetelet believed that the causal explanation of human behaviour could be found in antecedent and coexistent conditions, and if these were corrected, human behaviour would be improved. Florence Nightingale argued that if the conditions *causing* ill health, such as unclean water, inadequate sewage disposal and poor housing could be removed mankind would become healthy and, as she was later to put it, we could

'look to the abolition of all hospitals and workhouse infirmaries.'

to Henry Bonham Carter, June 1867

At the same time she fervently believed that she was called to 'dedicate her life to the Service of Mankind and that Service could only be rendered with the sanction of Service to God'. She pondered on the 'character of God' and she saw what she called God's law as the law of nature. It is noticeable that in *Notes on Nursing* she refers to disease as being '*A reparative process which nature has instituted*'. It is therefore the duty of the nurse to put the patient in a position for nature (that is God's law) to act on him.

It is this link with the statistical approach and the observation of God's law that is the matrix of Florence Nightingale's three volumes on religion, *Suggestions for Thought*. Originally written when she was 32 years old, it was dedicated to 'The Artizans of England and Seekers after Truth' who, she thought, were being led into error and atheism by the teachings of the Positivist, Auguste Comte, who maintained that 'all valid knowledge was based on verifiable fact and that precluded verifiable religion.'

Although she sets out her methodology clearly, Florence Nightingale's theological speculations are often difficult to follow, but their essence can be summed up in her own words:

'Granted that we see signs of universal law all over this world ie. law or plan or constant sequences in moral and intellectual, as well as physical phenomena of the world – granted this we must, in this universal law find traces of the Being who made it, and what is more of the *character* of the Being who made it. If we stop at the superficial signs, the Being is something so bad as no human character can be found to equal in badness, and certainly all beings He has made are better than himself.

But go deeper and see wider, and it appears as if this plan of *universal law* were the only one by which a good Being could teach His creatures to teach themselves and one another what is the road to universal perfection. And this we shall acknowledge is the only way for any educator, whether human or divine, to act – viz. to teach men to teach themselves and one another. If we could not *depend* upon God, ie. if this sequence were not always to be calculated upon in moral as well as in physical things – if He were to have caprices (by some called Grace, by others *answers to prayers* etc.) there would be no order in creation to depend upon. There would be chaos. And the only way by which man can have Free Will. ie. can learn to govern his own will, to have what he thinks right (which is having his will free), is to have universal Order or Law (by some miscalled Necessity) . . .

Philosophers have generally said that Necessity and Free Will are incompatible. It seems to have appeared to God that Law is the only way, on contrary, to give man his free will.'

to her father, July 1859
(Quoted in Cook [1], p. 482. Note that
when Miss Nightingale uses the second
person 'we' she is referring to herself,
and possible collaborators.)

Aunt Mai, who was looking after Miss Nightingale at that time, appears to have sent Mr Nightingale Volume 1 of *Suggestions for Thought*.

From this reasoning Florence Nightingale argues that God's scheme for us was not that he would give us what we asked for but that 'mankind should obtain it for mankind'. It is absurd to pray that God will alter his laws: they are the laws of nature and are unalterable. We know that if we eat deadly nightshade we will perish. We do not ask God to alter his laws to prevent it. We should not pray to God to be delivered from cholera, instead we should bend our efforts to provide a clean water supply for all citizens. It does not appear to have occurred to Florence Nightingale that we might pray to God to help us provide clean water, and, as Cranmer put it that 'we might know what things we ought to do'. It is interesting that in her theological exegesis Florence Nightingale takes a number of examples from what she called 'sanitary science'. It is no wonder that Lytton Strachey said that she saw God as 'a glorified Sanitary Engineer'.

Because God's laws are unalterable, Florence Nightingale sees the theory of forgiveness and absolution as untenable. How do we know when we are forgiven? This led her into difficulties with the Lord's Prayer, about which she had thought long and hard. As early as 1848 she had written to her father about the problem of human forgiveness, saying that she had come to the conclusion that forgiveness of others had to evolve. First, we had to learn to forgive, then we had to see that we had no business to be angry in the first place, there was, in fact, nothing to forgive. God whose understanding is complete, cannot forgive. He is impossible to offend. From this rationale she finds the Anglican theory of absolution confused. Could it be that this attitude to forgiveness ties up with Quetelet, in that human behaviour is affected by social conditions and, if we understand these, there is nothing to forgive?

The fact that God's laws are unalterable raises the question of a belief in miracles. She argued that because the will of God was expressed as an unalterable law, miracles, violations or interruptions of the law have no place in His scheme. In this she was influenced by the philosophies of Spinoza and the German intellectuals. She looked to the day when we would all feel as St Teresa and St Paul without recourse to miracles. She was certain that St Teresa did *not* see two little devils sitting on the priest's shoulder and that St Paul did *not* see a light in the sky; but she is sure that they, and other visionaries, believed what they saw and that it affected their lives.

The same belief in progress to 'perfectablity' underlies Florence Nightingale's eschatology. Each individual is unique, and it would be inconsistent with God's benevolent plan to extinguish that being. Therefore death must entail a different existence in which we move towards the perfect. This is a philosophy with which she was familiar from her studies of Plato, who, in Part XI of *The Republic*, argues that the soul is immortal because its own specific faults and moral wickedness cannot destroy it [2]. This was a belief held by a number of nineteenth-century poets and scholars, often leading to the concept of reincarnation.

Imbued with the spirit of Spinoza and the rationality of Comte, Florence Nightingale set out to refute the seventeenth-century philosopher John Locke, when he wrote

'We should prevail on the busy mind of man to be more cautious in meddling with things that exceed its comprehension, to stop when it is at the utmost of its tether and sit down in quiet ignorance of things that are beyond its capacity.' [3]

Florence Nightingale claimed that this philosophy had led people into error, but now her generation was wiser and was

determined to seek NO truth except that what is supposed to admit of truth.

Although she had set out to challenge Positivism, here we see Florence Nightingale coming close to Auguste Comte and, at the same time, the influence of Quetelet in the idea that social science and engineering will enable us to explain all phenomena and mankind will move towards 'perfectibility'. It was this unbounded optimism and the Victorian faith in steady human progress that led to the label 'The Whig interpretation of History' [4]. Over a hundred years later, after two horrendous world wars and the holocaust, we would question such optimism. Hubris was followed by Nemesis.

Suggestions for Thought were first written before Florence Nightingale went to the Crimea. Unlike most of her other prose which, though not elegant, is usually concise and littered with acerbic wit, this work is often prolix, repetitious and lacking in focus. If the Artizans of England ever read those 829 pages it is doubtful whether their faith would have been restored. Benjamin Jowett, a radical thinker to whom Arthur Clough, Florence Nightingale's poet cousin by marriage, sent a copy, turned it down as being 'full of antagonism'. Monckton Milnes commented that he 'did not think an omnipotent and implacable law any more satisfactory than a benevolent deity'. One suspects that Monckton Milnes, the champion of Keats, found it chilling. Julius von Mohl wrote, 'Florence set out to give the working class a religion, she gave them a philosophy instead'. The only approval came from John Stuart Mill, and this was probably because volume two is a diatribe about the subjection of women and is really out of place in a work on theology.

Florence Nightingale's combative tone about all contemporary religion, particularly the Church of England, is unduly harsh. Not all churchgoers found their churches 'cold and ugly', and for many it was a source of comfort in this troubleous life with its high mortality rate. Florence Nightingale had put away literary pursuits as 'a vain temptation'; she cared only for writing as a means to action. She did not see literary style as a means of influencing thought on a difficult subject, metaphor and allegory were lost on her and the beauty of the prose of the King James' Bible or Cranmer's prayers meant nothing to her in her obsession with tilting at biblical fundamentalism. Again, her contempt for parish charity and women 'trying to do a little good and doing a great deal of harm' ignores the fact that Victorian charity, though sometimes misguided, was the foundation of societies like The Society for the Prevention of Cruelty to Children and various groups of workers for people like the blind and the cripples, which were later the foundation for legislation and the welfare state.

Another problem arising from the philosophy that the adjustment of social conditions and the application of sanitary science would lead to a healthy population lies in the fact that good sanitation, however desirable, is not the panacea for all ills, and longevity itself produces its own health problems. Furthermore, scientific advance has its own side effects, some of which, like pollution, are deterimental and others, like nuclear fallout, lethal.

After deep searching and 'having learnt to know God', where did Florence Nightingale stand? She did not return to Unitarianism as some suggest, though this background was probably the mainspring of her doubts. She followed the controversy in the Victorian Church closely, the clash between Darwin and Wilberforce and the efforts of Churchmen like Jowett, Temple and Pattison to bridge the gap between Christian doctrine and the beliefs of educated men. This resulted in what came to be known as the 'Broad Church', a name coined by Arthur Clough, in which she eventually found a haven in her own idiosyncratic way. It is interesting that she became acquainted with Frederick Dennison Maurice, a friend of Bunsen, who consulted her, and who, like Clough, had lost his academic post because of his controversy over the sacraments. Maurice became a Christian Socialist and had ideas on social reform that were very much in tune with her own and who was to influence Beatrice Potter (later Mrs Webb).

Florence Nightingale's attitude to different creeds, and indeed different religions, was broadminded. This tolerance was manifest in the Nightingale School, which was for 'any class and any creed'. She had no time for religiosity for its own sake and certainly not for nurses 'who put their Bible work before the care of the sick'. For her the test of religion was to live it.

God

'What do we* mean by "God"? All we can say is that we recognise a power superior to our own; that we recognise that this power is exercised by a wise and good will.'

Suggestions for Thought, Vol. 1

On God's Law

'A law may be kept in various modes . . . The Law of gravity is kept whether a man falls down a precipice or stands on the earth . . . Our experience is that such laws are never broken. Thou shalt do no murder is broken many times in nineteenth century England. To call it a volition of God is to say that God's will is NOT always done.'

ibid., Vol. 3

The Ten Commandments

'Are they not full of mistakes?
    The 5th. 1. We can only honour what is honourable
            2. Filial piety has nothing to do with living to an old age
            3. The Lord did not give them the land. (in the sense that Moses said)
            They took it.'

ibid., Vol. 1

The Scriptures

'Men do not read the Bible because their commonsense resists such things as *"take nothing for your journey, neither scrip nor staff, neither bread nor money* . . . " Things that belong to the Esserne communities, not these . . . Men cannot bear these things, yet will be shocked at not thinking Christ divine. We too think him divine, but not the *only* divine one.'

ibid., Vol. 1

Prayer

'We are destitute of the first principles of knowledge with regard to God's nature His plans with man, his manner . . . If we prayed that an eclipse set down in our almanac would not take place would this be more absurd than praying that one of God's moral laws should be altered?'

ibid., Vol. 1

* 'We' in *Suggestions for Thought* refers to Florence Nightingale.

'If He [God] were changed by people praying to Him we would be at the mercy of all who prayed to Him.'

Private note, 18[??]

'Many believed that cholera was traceable to no other origin than the direct will of a super human power . . . the means attempted to prevent it were prayer which it was hoped would influence God's will, or some changing circumstance, totally irrelevant to the case.'

Suggestions for Thought, Vol. 1
(Although Florence Nightingale appreci-
ated that cholera was a disease that
flourished in poor hygiene, i.e. poor san-
itary conditions, she never accepted the
germ theory.)

Miracles

'People are terrified of religion without miracles and belief in miracles certainly makes them happy . . . but what a lowering of the conception of God.'

ibid., Vol. 2

'Did God speak to us? There is hardly anything which it is supposed that God did say than which we could not have thought of for ourselves.'

ibid., Vol. 1
(Florence Nightingale always claimed
that God had spoken to her twice in her
life.)

Sin

'Did this man sin or his parents? That question implied a false idea . . . Sin regards those laws only which concern our spiritual and moral being, that is our feelings towards God and our fellow creatures. That a man is blind implies some ignorance of physical law either on his own part or on those who preceded him.'

ibid., Vol. 1

Forgiveness

'God cannot forgive. His laws have assigned consequents entirely definite to every antecedent . . . Neither can we pray that he will alter the laws of perfect goodness and wisdom with regard to spiritual things. We would not be perfect if he did.'

ibid., Vol. 3

The Church Of England

'The Church of England has men for bishoprics, archbishoprics, and a little work
. . . For women she has – what? have no taste for theological discoveries. I would
have given her my head, my hand, my heart. She would not have them. She did
not know what to do with them. She told me to go back and do crochet in my
mother's drawing room; or if I were tired of that to marry and look well at the
head of my husband's table. You may go to Sunday School if you like, she said.
But she gave me no training for that . . . She gave neither work to do for her nor
education for it.'

Letter to Dr Stanley, October 1852

'We believe that *all* the faculties of mankind should be exercised to receive
the revelation of God to man. The Anglicans and the Roman Catholics etc etc
etc exercise a limited number of faculties in what they receive as revelation.'

Suggestions for Thought, Vol. 1

'Does the Church look like an assemblage of men fitted to find out religious
truth?'

ibid.

Misguided Giving

'People go to Church, teach their children the catechism and creed and give away
flannel petticoats and broth which is called "doing good" . . . But now it is truly
said of many a woman "she has been trying all her life to do a little good and
has done a great deal of harm". People know that giving away is not doing good,
yet they do not know what to put in its place.'

ibid.

*(Florence Nightingale was unduly hard on the Church of England and its oppor-
tunities for women. The Oxford Movement saw the founding of a number of orders
where women did not take vows but worked in hospitals, in the community and in
teaching. These included the Sisters of St John, from whom Florence Nightingale
learned much about nursing [5], the Sisters of All Saints and the Sellonites from
Plymouth who provided nurses for the Crimea. All provided some training.)*

The Church Of Rome

'You do know now, with all its faults, what a Home the Catholic Church is. And
yet what she is to you compared with what she would be to me? No one can
tell what she is to women. What training is there (in the Church of England)
compared with that of the Catholic nun. Why cannot I enter the Catholic Church

at once, as the best form of truth I have ever known, and as cutting the Gordian knot I cannot untie?'

to Cardinal Manning, July 1852
(Manning converted to Rome in 1850.)

Unitarians and Trinitarians

'Unitarians say no man is divine, none an incarnation of God: the Trinitarians say one (who was divine). What do we mean by a man being divine or an incarnation of God? Are not all men "incarnations of God"? . . . Trinitarianism is a truer doctrine than Unitarianism.'

Suggestions for Thought, Vol. 1

'We make a distinction almost similar [to the religion of ancient Egypt] between Father, Son and the Holy Ghost (if I may say so) the hand ie. the worker, the communicating medium . . . '

Letters from Egypt, 1854

Evangelicals

' . . . So often complain of their hard hearts (Wesley's whole tone is nothing else) they say they cannot love God. Is it any wonder? How can they love a being they only imagine. They work themselves up by excitement into a spasm of interest about Him, but they must find their hearts hard to a religion so essentially cold.'

Suggestions for Thought, Vol. 1

Holy Communion

'God communicates with us by His nature actually becoming ours. The Roman Catholic, who sincerely believes that he eats the body and drinks the blood of Him in whom God manifested himself – well may he feel himself invigorated, ennobled, penetrated! What grand ideas: grand because true, are these of Divine manifestations in the human, of the Divine received into but becoming human . . . '

ibid., Vol. 1

(Florence Nightingale had little interest in the rites of the Church as such, but she found comfort in the sacrament of Holy Communion; while she was an invalid, Jowett often came up from Oxford to administer it to her and she was sometimes joined by members of her family, who were a closer unit than we are often led to suppose.)

Belief In Progress

'The history of human nature is the history of progress, or the preparation of progress towards feelings and manifestations that we distinguish as MORAL right and righteousness. God's law is such that the history of men is tending to bring about such feelings in human nature.'

ibid., Vol. 3

Life After Death

'To suppose that each individual does contribute his portion then retires from existence to make room for others is inconsistent with the spirit of love and wisdom. It is true that something is transmitted to another generation, but experience shows that no mode of existence is wasted or destroyed. It is all evolution, development, order, progress – never destruction.

He will realise the full perfect development which is His thought, though it requires ages beyond the grasp of our minds to conceive.'

ibid., Vol. 3

'I am sure it is an immense activity.'

Reply to Lady Stephen (William Shore's daughter) who had suggested that the afterlife was 'being at rest', 1900

Under Church Of Rome

' . . . And now I do feel that it is the strength of our country and worth all the R Catholic "Orders" put together . . . I hate an "Order" & am so glad I was never "let in" to form one.'

to Samuel Smith (her financial adviser), 1861
(On the death of a self-taught man who had been one of her 'pupils' in sanitary engineering.)

Doubts

'Not even my "pupils" would take anything from me if they knew I read Spinoza. One of them wrote to me 12 pages beginning: "How is it that no one denies your philanthrophy, every one doubts your Christianity?" To which I replied with the utmost sincerity, that she was quite right in thinking me a very poor follower of Christ.'

to Benjamin Jowett, 1865
(The pupil was Agnes Jones, an Irish Presbyterian.)

'Sometimes I ask myself, after all my "Laws" & "Moral Worlds," is there a God after all?'

to Julius von Mohl, 1873
(On the sufferings in India.)

On the Revision of the Old and New Testaments

'Also in St Paul's Conversion: they have omitted those memorable words which have saved so many.

"Lord, what wilt Thou have me to do?"

How short the prayers in the N T are: how heart felt.'

to Edmund Verney, 1897

References

[1] Cook Sir E (1913) *The Life of Florence Nightingale*, Vol. 1, p. 482. *London: Macmillan*.

[2] Plato (427–347 B.C.) *The Republic*, p. 442. Penguin Classics.

[3] Locke J (1690) *Essay Concerning Human Understanding*.

[4] Butterfield H (1931) *The Whig Interpretation of History*. Reprinted Pelican, 1973, pb.

[5] Baly M E (1986) *Florence Nightingale and the Nursing Legacy*, p. 67 ff. London: Croom Helm.

4

Of Wars and Armies

Although Florence Nightingale is popularly associated with the Crimean War (1854–6), she was earlier passionately interested in the politics of Europe and the revolutions of 1848. The Crimea gave her an almost mystical devotion to the Army and its welfare, and thereafter she followed avidly the campaigns in the British Empire, including Africa and India, with a particular interest in the Egyptian campaigns and the Boer War when she advised on the sending of nurses. In her letters to probationers she was fond of comparing the discipline of nurses to the discipline of the Army. Although deeply disturbed by the horror of war, Florence Nightingale could never be classed as a pacifist and was ambivalent about 'war bringing out the best'.

Miss Nightingale and her party of thirty-eight nurses left for Scutari on 21 October 1854, a week after receiving a letter from Sidney Herbert. She remained there with various groups of nurses, who tended to come and go, until July 1856.

The story of the appalling unpreparedness of the Army Medical Services for the casualties of the war is well documented, as is Miss Nightingale's battle with officialdom. The main lesson she learned about nursing was how to steer between the 'Protestant Howl and the Roman Catholic Storm'; the Crimea convinced her that nursing must be non-sectarian. But the overriding message from her letters is that she sees, rightly, that much of the suffering was preventable. No fewer than 17,600 soldiers died of disease. Miss Nightingale's contribution to suffering humanity was not in introducing female nurses to the Army Medical Service, but in hammering home the message that many of the casualties had been preventable. 'I stand at the altar of murdered men and while I live I will fight their cause' was to be her battle-cry when she returned to England. Her letters home show how she hated the 'fuzz-buzz' about her name and the fear that it would detract from the main purpose. She had the remarkable sense to see that being a national heroine would do nothing to help reform the Army Medical Service. At the same time, it is interesting to notice that, hard-pressed and almost hysterical as she was at times, she never lost her talent for purple prose and the carefully thought-out alliteration. Small wonder that people kept her letters.

On Return from the Crimea

Florence Nightingale returned from the Crimea in July 1856 and for the next year she worked feverishly trying to get a Royal Commission of Enquiry into the defects of the Army Medical Service and the soldier's life in general. With the aid of the doctors and engineers she had met in the Crimea and of men like the statistician William Farr, she made herself an expert on the best sanitation of the day and on barrack construction. Now her abiding passion was *not* to reform nursing or provide worthwhile careers for women but to prevent unnecessary deaths and ill health both in military hospitals and in civilian life.

Then, on 11th August 1857, she collapsed and it was thought she would die; her obituary notices were brought up to date. At that stage she probably wanted to die. The cause and course of her illness has been the subject of much, and at times bizarre, speculation. When she returned from the Crimea her emaciated appearance and agitated state were the results of the attack of 'Crimean Fever' in 1855, which was most likely Brucella melitensis [1] which tends to have long term sequelae and cause personality changes. The primary reason why Miss Nightingale took to her bed, or couch, is that is what the doctors ordered, it was standard practice for cardiac dysfunction. It was also accepted medical wisdom that excessive mental exertion by a woman was abnormal and would lead to a breakdown. From then on it is difficult to separate her symptoms, which she often describes vividly in letters, from the treatment she received, including bed rest, isolation from social contact, and drugs, including opium needles and bromides. Apart from the iatrogenic element there was consciously, or unconsciously, a psychosomatic element. As T. S. Eliot said, referring to himself and other eminent writers who experienced 'breakdowns', 'it is commonplace that some forms of illness are extremely valuable to artistic and literary composition' [2]. Miss Nightingale now found that 'last letters' concentrated minds and spurred action. Not for her was the wasting of time outside in the corridors of power. From now on they came to her, and by appointment. Whether or not there was an organic reason for the nearly 20 years as an invalid we will never know, we should take John Locke's advice (p.23) and 'sit down in quiet ignorance'.

What is important is that from her bed she now made her great contribution to the health and welfare of the Army, who probably owe her a greater debt than does nursing; to the collection of medical statistics; to hospital building; to the sanitation in India and the Poor Law infirmaries in England; and lastly, and perhaps less importantly, because she was not alone in this field, the reform of midwifery and nursing services. One thing is certain: to her dying day her Crimean experience and the harsh lot of the British soldier, whose cause she never ceased to champion, remained written on her heart.

Of Wars and Armies

'They must carry on their defence to the last. I should like to see them fight in the streets inch by inch till the last man dies at his barricade, till St Peter's is levelled to the ground, till the Vatican is blown in the air . . . Michael Angelo would cry "Well done" as he saw his work destroyed.'

to Mme Mohl, April 1848, Rome
(During the winter spent in Rome with
the Bracebridges (q.v.), Miss Nightingale
saw something of the Italian revolution.)

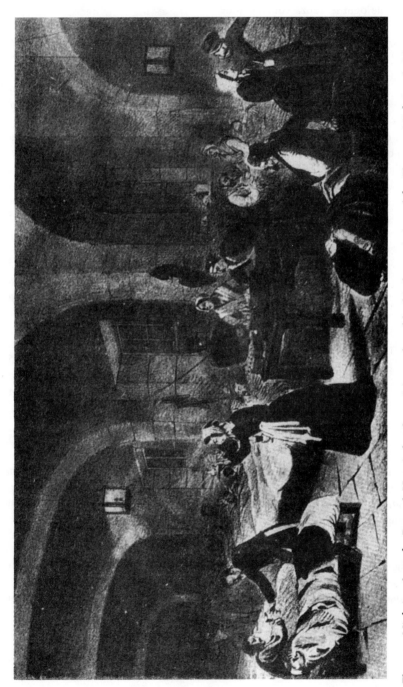

Florence Nightingale at the Barrack Hospital at Scutari (reproduced by kind permission of the Florence Nightingale Museum Trust).

'Lasciate ogni speranza voi ch'entrate.'

> *('Abandon hope all ye that enter here,' 5*
> *November 1854 from Dante's Divine*
> *Comedy, Canto III, which Miss*
> *Nightingale said should be written over*
> *the doorway of the Barrack Hospital,*
> *Scutari.)*

'But oh! you gentlemen of England who sit at Home in the well-earned satisfaction of your successful cases, can have little idea from reading your newspapers of the Horror and Misery of operating on these dying and exhausted men. A London hospital is a garden of flowers to it.'

> *to Dr William Bowman, 14 November*
> *1854*

'The strongest will be wanted to the wash tub.'

> *3 November 1854*
> *(To the nurse who said: 'When we land*
> *don't let there be any red tape, let us get*
> *straight to nursing the poor fellows.')*

'Calamity unparalleled in the history of calamity.'

> *to Sidney Herbert, 4 January 1855*
> *(With 12,000 men in hospital and more*
> *still pouring in.)*

'Nursing is the least of the functions into which I have been forced.'

> *to Sidney Herbert, 8 January 1855*

'I am a kind of general dealer in socks, shirts, knives and forks, wooden spoons, tin baths, tables and forms, cabbages and carrots, operating tables, towels and soap, small tooth combs, precipitate for destroying lice, scissors, bedpans and stump pillows.'

> *to Sidney Herbert, 3 January 1855*

'The Commission has done nothing . . . Canning has done nothing, Lord Wm Paulet has done nothing, Lord Stratford, absorbed in politics, does not know the circumstances, Lord Wm Paulet knows them but partially, Menzies knows them all and will not tell them, Wreford knows them and is stupefied. The Medical Officers, if they were to betray them, would have it "reported personally and professionally to their disadvantage" . . . '

> *to Sidney Herbert, 8 January 1855*

'I never look at *The Times*, but they tell me there is a religious war about poor me there, and that Mrs H has generously defended me. I do not know what I have done to be so dragged before the Public. But I am so glad that my God is not the God of the High Church or of the Low, that he is not a Romanist or an Anglican or a Unitarian. I don't believe he is even a Russian – tho' his events go strangely against us. A Greek once said to me on Salamis "I do believe God Almighty is an Englishman".'

> *to Sidney Herbert, 28 January 1855*
> *(The religious conflict was due to the*
> *party brought out by Mary Stanley,*
> *where Mother Bridgeman decreed it was*
> *the nurses' duty to minister to the*
> *spiritual needs of the Irish soldiers; this*
> *was against the original agreement with*
> *the Government and with Manning.*
> *When Miss Nightingale tried to*
> *intervene, she was accused of being like*
> *'Herod sending the Blessed Virgin*
> *across the desert'.)*

'A great deal has been said of our self-sacrifice, heroism and so forth. The real humiliation, the real hardship of this place, dear Mr Herbert, is that we have to do with men who are neither gentlemen, nor men of education, nor even men of business, nor men of feeling, but [men] whose only object is to keep out of blame.'

> *to Sidney Herbert, February 1855*

'What the horrors of war are no one can imagine. They are not the wounds and the blood and the fever-spotted and low – dysentery – chronic and acute – and cold and heat and famine. They are intoxication, drunken brutality, demoralisation and disorder on the part of the inferior; jealousies, meanness and indifference, selfish brutality on the part of the superior.'

> *to Sidney Herbert, May 1855*

'I hope you are doing something about the Monument. Please put yourself *at once* in communication, dear Pop, with the Chaplain General Gleig to get up working drawings for our public monument and private chapel now to be enclosed on a cliff looking over the Sea of Marmora . . .

As for myself, I have done my duty. I have identified my fate with that of the heroic dead and whatever lies these sordid exploiters of human misery spread about us these officials, there is a right and a God to fight for and our fight has been worth fighting. I do not despair – nor complain. It has been a great cause.'

> *To Parthenope, 8 March 1855*

'Please date your letters.'

> *(F.N. often did not date hers!)*

'The camp [Balaclava] is very striking, more so than one can imagine or describe ... But to me the most affecting sight was to see them [the soldiers] mustering and forming fours at sun down for the trenches where they will be for 24 hours without returning. From those trenches 30 will never return. Yet they volunteer – press forward for the trenches. When I consider what the work has been this winter, what the hardships, I am surprised – not that the army has suffered so much but – that there is any army left at all . . .

It is a wonderful sight looking down on Sevastopol – the shell whizzing right and left. I send you a Minié bullet I picked up on the ground which was ploughed with shot and shell and some little flowers.'

to Parthenope, 10 May 1855, Balaclava

'The vanity and frivolity which the éclat thrown upon this affair has called forth has done us unmitigated harm and brought forth mischief on perhaps the most promising enterprise that ever set out from England [the Nursing Party]. The small still beginning, the simple hardship, the silent *gradual* struggle upwards, this is the climate in which enterprise really grows and thrives.'

to Parthe, July 1855

'A little gin would be more popular.'

[?] October 1855 (Scribbled note on hearing that Queen Victoria had offered to send the troops eau de cologne)

'I have been appointed a 12 month today and what a 12 month of dirt it has been, of experience that would sadden not life but eternity. Who has ever had a sadder experience? Christ was betrayed by one but my cause has been betrayed by everyone, alas one may truly say excepting Mrs Roberts, Rev. Mother and Mrs Stewart. All the rest, Weare, Clough, Salisbury, Stanley *et id, genus omne*, where are they?'

to Aunt Mai, 5 November 1855

'There is not an official who would not burn me like Joan of Arc if he could, but they know that the War Office cannot turn me out because the country is with me. That is the position.'

to Sidney Herbert, November 1855

'Everything, I believe I may say *everything* was done either on earth or under the earth to make me resign during the Crimean War. But I never felt a moment's doubt on the question:
I would not resign.
I might be driven from my post.
I would not run away.'

to Rachel Williams (who was threatening to resign), 2 December 1884

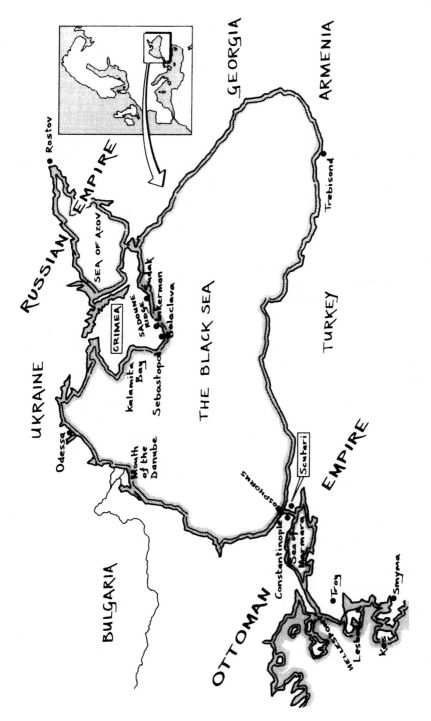

Map of the Black Sea at the time of the Crimean War.

'My reputation has not been a boon to my work, but if you have been pleased it is enough.'

to Mrs Nightingale, December 1855
(On hearing about the public meeting at
Willis's Rooms to inaugurate the
Nightingale Fund, 29 November 1855.)

'The real grievance against us is that we are independent of promotion and therefore of the great displeasure of our Chiefs – that we have no prospects to injure – & that, altho' subordinate to these Medical Chiefs in office, we are superior to them in influence & in the chance of being heard at home. It is an anomalous position. But so is war, to us English, anomalous.'

to Elizabeth Herbert, 17 November
1855, Balaclava

' . . . Nurses [in Military Hospitals] must not be under the *immediate* direction of the Principal Medical Officer . . . I have never had the slightest difficulty about this – tho Medical Men always coming to me saying "I want such and such assistance" – and I am always informing them of any exchange or removal of Nurses – & consulting them. But I would never have undertaken the Superintendency with that condition that the Nurses consider themselves "under the direction of the Principal Medical Officer". I am under his direction. *They* are under mine.'

to Lady Canning, September 1853
(Here Florence Nightingale emphatically
lays down the chain of command and the
accountability of nurses; this was to
become the sine qua non *of her reforms,*
and the cause of many battles then and
later.)

'I do not presume to express praise or gratitude to you Rev'd Mother, because it would look as if I thought you had done the work not unto God but to me. You were far above me in fitness for the General Superintendency – both in worldly talent of administration and far more in spiritual qualifications which God values in a superior.'

to Rev'd Mother Clare Moore, April
1856
('Mother Bermondsey' was going home
because of ill health, having borne most
of the trials and hardships that Scutari
could throw at her.)

'During these ten days . . . I have never been off my horse till 9 or 10 at night when it was too dark to walk him over the crags . . . During the greater part of the day I have been without food except for a little brandy (you see I am taking to drink like my comrades in the Army). But the object has been obtained and my women [the nurses in the Crimea] have neither starved nor suffered.'

to Sidney Herbert, April 1856
(Reporting on her visit to the hospitals
in the Crimea. This is part of a long
letter in which she sets out the
deficiences in purveying and
administration. Officialdom had hit back
at her interference and Sidney Herbert
needed all his 'angelic patience' to deal
with the different factions.)

'I can fire my own guns.'

to Dr Farr, 1856
(Recollected by Mary Farr years later.)

'My Lord is, as I have often found, the most bullyable of mortals.'

to Sidney Herbert, December 1856
(Note on her interview with
Lord Panmure, Secretary of State
for War.)

'Give them opportunity promptly & securely to send money home – & they will use it.

Give them a school and a lecture and they will come to it.

Give them a book & a game & a magic Lanthorn & they will leave off drinking.

Give them suffering and they will bear it.

Give them work and they will do it.

I would rather have to do with the army generally than with any other class I have ever attempted to serve.'

to Lt Col. J. H. Lefroy, 6 March 1856
(On the ordinary soldier.)

'The way to improve the soldier's morals is to improve his living conditions.'

to Edwin Chadwick, 1862

'I am a bad mother to come home and leave you in your Crimean graves, 73 per cent in 8 regiments in six months from disease alone – who thinks of that now?'

Private note, July 1856

'No one can feel for the Army as I do. These people who talk to us have all fed their children on the fat of the land and dressed them in velvet and silk while we have been away. I have had to see my children dressed in a dirty blanket and an old pair of regimental trowsers, and to see them fed on raw salt meat, and nine thousand of my children are lying from causes, which might have been prevented, in their forgotten graves. But I can never forget. People must have seen that long dreadful winter to know what it was.'

Private note, 9 February 1857

'Dear Mr Herbert,
I received your letter of 6th March yesterday. It is written from Belgrave Square. I write from a Crimean Hut. The point of sight is different.
    [*There follow pages of the difficulties and obstructions to the work in the Crimea and Scutari.*]
    But all I wish to leave is some record of what will not be believed in the homes of London a twelvemonth hence – of what, tho' a trifling instance, is a true example of what ruined our Army . . . '

to Sidney Herbert, 3 April 1856

'Nous avons rien oublié ni rien appris. . . . In six months all this suffering will be forgotten.'

Private note, April 1856 ('We have
forgotten nothing and learnt nothing';
on hearing of the declaration of peace.)

'If I could only carry *one* point which would prevent *one* part of the recurrence of the colossal calamity; then I should be true to the brave dead.'

Private note, August 1856

'I stand at the altar of murdered men.'

Private note, 1856 and 1857

'The publicity and talk there has been about this work have injured it more than anything else, and in no way, I am determined will I contribute by making a show of myself.'

Private note, August 1856
(On refusing receptions and
presentations on her return to England.)

'Father, I do not in the least care whether I live or die. I would wish to know what it is to be, that I may know what thou wouldst have of me. I do not suppose there will be any less work for us in any future state of existence. Wilt Thou send us where most work is wanted to be done . . . '

Private note, August 1857
(In August, Florence Nightingale was
expected to die within weeks.)

'I Hope you will not regret the manner of my death. I know you will be kind enough to regret the fact of it.
. . .

I am sorry about the Nursing scheme [the Nightingale Fund] It seems like leaving it in the lurch. Mrs Shaw Stewart is the only woman I know who will do for Supt, of Army Nurses.'

to Sidney Herbert, November 1857
(Florence Nightingale had clearly given
the Nightingale Fund no thought since
her return. Mrs Shaw Stewart, a well
educated lady with considerable
experience had run a hospital in the
Crimea [3].)

'My God, My God why hast thou forsaken us.'

Private note [?], 1857
(At this stage it looked as if there would
be a whitewashing report and the whole
tragedy forgotten. In the end the
Commission made some progress largely
due to her persistence.)

'We came home, with the remains of the lost Army to see the Throne taking to its bosom the most distinguished of the malefactors . . . And what do we remember of these men in past tragedy? . . .

Words were given in plenty, to the great Crimean catastrophe. But the real tragedy began when it was over. The great town proprietors in England send about broth and blue frocks, but they let people in their houses live in a condition that leaves the impossibility of health, of morality, or even domestic affection . . . there was no Poor Law, no market for labour, no trade or commerce . . . these people starved . . . '

Extract from a long and bitter private
note, 1857
(On the social and economic conditions
for the underclass in Victorian England.
It is the cry of returning soldiers down
the ages.)

'The words you use about your health are also, as far as I have been able to learn, applicable, word for word, to mine, which I only mention to show that I too have "no future" and must do what I can without delay.'

to Harriet Martineau, December 1856
(Harriet Martineau had been diagnosed
as terminally ill, though later she rose
from her bed and lived to the age of 74
years. She was the recipient of
Florence's 'confidential leaks' to the
press. Although they disagreed on a
number of matters, Harriet remained a
good ally.)

'Official whitewash.'

(Note on Mr Mellor's report of the
purveying at Scutari, 1857.)

'Reports are not Self-Executive.'

(Written in the margin of the Royal
Sanitary Commission Report, July 1858,
and repeated several times in private
notes.)

'I am being worked on a treadmill.'

to Sidney Herbert, July 1858 (On
preparing the evidence to the
Commission.)

'The War Office is a very slow and enormously expensive office.'

to Sidney Herbert, 1858

'You might as well take 1,000 men every year out upon Salisbury Plain and shoot them.'

On the State of the Barracks in England,
Miss Nightingale's evidence to the
Commission, 1858

'There are rats in the W.O. – also a cat. There are 17 months of minutes to apply for 6d a week for her, 40 minutes to say that she ought to live on rats. Other minutes to say she ought to have milk but that 6d a week is too much. Others ask what she is to live on in the mean time. I am very anxious to know your decision, whether you have given one yet, whether you think 5¾ too much. I incline to 5½.'

to Sidney Herbert, October 1860
(In the Herbert papers at Wilton.)

'I am exceedingly anxious to see your charming gift, especially those returns showing Deaths, Admissions and Diseases.'

to Dr William Farr December 1860
(The statistics were to be a New Year's
gift.)

'I must retrench.'

New Year resolution, 1861
(This tended to be recurring.)

'He [Sidney Herbert] has not one cardinal symptom of confirmed disease. . . . There is no proof that he has organic disease other than incipient. . . . Almost all physicians are quacks.'

to Liz Herbert, 14 May 1861
(Three months before Sidney Herbert
died, having been gravely ill with kidney
disease for two years.)

'My work, the object of my life, the means to do it all depart with him.'

to Mr Nightingale, August 1861

'I was too hard on him . . . but at the same time he knew what I said was true.'

to Harriet Martineau, September 1861

'This is the shortest day, would it were the last. Adieu dear friend. I am worse . . .
  I am glad to end a day which can never come again, gladder to end the night, gladder still to end a month.'

to Mary Clarke, December 1861
(1861 saw the deaths of Lord Herbert
and Arthur Clough, her poet cousin by
marriage and the first secretary of the
Nightingale Fund, and also the death of
the Prince Consort, whom she regarded
as an ally. She wished for death.)

'I have fought the good fight with the War Office and lost it.'

to Dr William Farr, 1861

'Agitate, Agitate.'

Telegram from Miss Nightingale to
Harriet Martineau, 1863
(That is, agitate for Lord de Grey to
succeed Sir George Lewis at the War
Office. Florence Nightingale was fighting
to keep a foot in the War Office and
carry on with Sidney Herbert's work.)

'I agree with you that it will be quite harmless for a government to sign the Convention as it now stands. It amounts to nothing more than a declaration that humanity to the wounded is a good thing. . . . Besides which though I do not reckon myself to be an inhumane person, I can conceive of circumstances of *force majeure* in war when the more people who are killed the better.'

to General Thomas Longmore, British
Representative at the Geneva
Convention, August 1864

'I do not know if Hamlet was mad but he would have driven me mad.'

to Mme Mohl, 1868
(On indecision in high places.)

'I am so overwhelmed with business that I must be brief. In 17 years I have had 2 weeks' holiday – excepting what God gave me in Typhus Fever in 1855. I was just going to take a third week – when this awful cloud of war* which darkens the world came over us. And all that *can* be, how little, *must* be done for the sufferers by one already overladen with business & an incurable illness. How willingly would I die to save any portion of this awful misery.'

to Mrs Cox, 7 August 1870
(Mrs Cox was the organiser of war relief
in northern France.)

'Few men, and fewer women have seen so much of the horrors of war as I have. Yet, I cannot say that war seems to me an unmitigated evil. The soldier in war is a *man*: devoted to his duty, giving his life for his comrade, his God. . . . Then would you always have war? Well, I have nothing to do with making war or peace. I can only say you must see a man in war to know what he is capable of. If you drive past a barracks you will see two heads idling and

---

*The Franco-Prussian War with which Miss Nightingale became closely involved. She had close friends in both France and Prussia. She consequently worked with the National Society for Aid to the Sick and Wounded and was awarded both the Bronze Cross by the French Société de Secours aux Blessés and the Prussian Cross of Merit by the Kaiser in 1871.

lolling out of every window . . . And the moral is: Provide the soldier with active employment.'

October 1899
(On the outbreak of the Boer War)

References

[1] *British Medical Journal* (1995) Volume 311, 23–30 December.
[2] Eliot T S (1975) in *Virginia Woolf: The Critical Heritage*, ed. Robin Majumda. London.
[3] Baly M E (1986) *Florence Nightingale and the Nursing Legacy*, Chapter 6. London: Routledge.

5

Social Policy

Early in her life, Florence Nightingale was convinced of the importance of preventive measures in social policies. During parish visiting with her mother and sister in the 1840s – the 'hungry forties' – she saw the effects of the industrial revolution on the changing employment opportunities for the poor and the fact that grinding poverty destroyed not only health 'but morality and domestic affection'. She would have agreed with Bernard Shaw when he wrote 'I can't preach religion to a man with hunger in his eyes' [1]. It is for this reason that she was so caustic about 'soup and flannel petticoat' charity: 'don't give a beggar alms, give him work' would have been her maxim.

Strongly influenced by Quetelet and the early sociologists (see Chapter 3), she believed that if such conditions as poverty, ignorance and poor living conditions could be changed, mankind's behaviour could be altered. Her attitude to the poor and the deprived, and to the British soldier, also stemmed from her profound belief that all men (and women) are fellow creatures to be nursed to health and all are capable of 'perfectibility'. In this Florence Nightingale is like Elizabeth Fry. She returned from the Crimea with the burning conviction that much illness was preventable and what was needed was a strong draught of sanitary science.

Overworked and ill though she was, it is for this reason that she lent a sympathetic ear to William Rathbone's plea for a training scheme for 'district nurses' in Liverpool. Contrary to the Ladies Committee who saw a nurse, duly controlled by them, to be a dispenser of charity, Miss Nightingale saw it as a service which would nurse and, at the same time, educate the poor sick and help them to return to work.

The greatest part of nineteenth century mortality and morbidity was due to water-borne and animal vector diseases, and although Miss Nightingale clung to the miasma theory well after the germ theory of infection had been established, by insisting on clean water and rigorous hygiene she was doing the right thing for the wrong reason. It is arguable that her contribution to public health and community care was greater than her contribution to the reform of hospital nursing, which would have come in any case as medicine became more scientific and the hospitals were used by the middle classes. Indeed, it could be contested that the so-called 'Nightingale System' was not necessarily the best paradigm for nursing education. However, the promotion of trained district nursing was invaluable and, later, so was the unique concept of training a separate corps of health visitors, whose work was to play an important part in the dramatic fall in the infant mortality rate and the improvement in the health of school children in the first part of the twentieth century.

The Poor Law

Because she was convinced that much poverty and its associated poor health was preventable, Miss Nightingale saw the punitive Poor Law Amendment Act of 1834 as wrongheaded. This Act, in order to reduce the cost of outdoor relief, had introduced the 'less eligibility test' where paupers were to be treated 'less favourably than the lowest paid labourer'. The result was that 'the sick, the old, the infirm and the mentally and physically disabled had been herded together in large Workhouses' [2]. Miss Nightingale was not alone in regarding the fate of the sick paupers as a disgrace; there was a strong Workhouse Reform Movement, but the reformers were divided between those who wanted to alleviate the lot of the paupers *within* the framework of the Act and those, like John Stuart Mill and Miss Nightingale, who wanted to abolish the Act and change the system.

Miss Nightingale's attitude on the need for the social services to be organised by a central authority is interesting in the light of subsequent history; she is foreshadowing William Beveridge and the Webbs and, later, the idea of a central health authority complete with a Central Bed Bureau. Most Victorians believed that society's ills could be cured by thrift, self-help and charity, maintaining that it was important that there should be a nexus between the giver of charity and the recipient. The recipient of course would be 'the worthy' or 'the deserving poor'. Miss Nightingale, like Mr Doolittle in Shaw's *Pygmalion*, did not differentiate between the two categories and her attitude to the problem of unemployment was almost Keynesian; it was up to the state to help create employment possibilities.

As far as the sick paupers were concerned, she argued that they should cease to be treated as paupers, i.e. made 'less eligible', and nursed back to health in conditions as good as in any civil hospital. This was, of course, anathema to the legislators who saw the 'workhouse test' as a deterrent to the able-bodied seeking relief. Miss Nightingale saw, as few did, that the great mass of paupers were the sick, the old and those handicapped in some way. The Nightingale Fund Council, to its credit, financed several experiments introducing trained nursing to Poor Law infirmaries [3]. The first was in Liverpool, which really ended in failure except that it provided nursing with a martyr, which was useful propaganda. The second was at Highgate (later Whittington hospital) and the third, and most successful, with Miss Vincent at St Marylebone. Other Nightingale nurses like Amy Hughes continued to carry the torch for trained nursing in workhouses, and by the end of the century it had become an accepted fact, though, sadly, the stigma attached to these institutions was to remain for a long time to come.

Penal Reform

As a disciple of Quetelet, Miss Nightingale was firmly of the belief that aberrant behaviour was produced by the effects of poor social and educational backgrounds;

if these could be removed, men would, in time, become morally improved (see Chapter 3). Therefore, incarceration in prison without attempt at reform was useless, it only made the situation worse. By the same logic she was firmly against capital punishment, arguing, as did Elizabeth Fry, that every person is a soul to be saved and death denies 'time for amendment of life'. By the same reasoning, sinners (even murderers) were often the product of their social environment; she denied the idea of eternal damnation and her Unitarian background led her to reject the doctrine of original sin, which put her at odds with most of the Church of England. She was in many ways ahead of her time on matters of social policy and, had she been born later, she would undoubtedly have been a member of the Howard League for Penal Reform.

Policy on India

During the 1860s and 1870s, Miss Nightingale spent a great deal of time researching the problems of sanitation in the Army in India; it was said that many of the files for the India Office were to be found at her house in South Street. Every Governor General of India came to see her before he left, and some, like Sir John Lawrence, became close friends. Never having been to India, she made mistakes on to which her detractors have fastened gleefully, but she was basically right about the importance of irrigation and the need for a pure water supply, and, unlike many of her class, she had a real sympathy for the Indian peasant and the Parsee, a sympathy that was akin to her feeling for the ordinary soldier.

Social Policy

'It is mere childishness to tell us that it is not important to know what houses people live in. . . . The connection between *health* and the dwellings of the population is one of the most important that exists.'

to Robert Lowe, 1861
(On the design of the Census form.)

'I wish my life were beginning. I think I could do something to inoculate the country with the view of preventing instead of "cure".'

to Douglas Galton, 1862

'I was much obliged to that poor man for dying. It was want of cleanliness. Mr Villiers says he will never hear the last of it in the H. of C.'

to Sir John McNeill, 7 February 1865
(On the death of Timothy Daly in the
Holborn Workhouse.)

'The only way to decrease venereal disease is to give the soldier more chances of respectable marriage, better housing and opportunities for recreation besides the public house.'

to Lord de Grey, Secretary of State for War, 1864

'Scarcely anything is so much wanted for civilization as an organization of this sort [the scheme to divide Liverpool into Districts, each with a "District Nurse"]. Scarcely in any other city in Europe is it so neglected as in London.'

to Henry Bonham Carter, June 1867

'To set poor people going again with a sound and clean house as well as a sound body and mind is about as great a benefit as can be given them – worth acres of relief. This is depauperizing them.'

to William Rathbone, 1867

'So long as a sick man, woman or child is considered administratively to be a pauper to be *repressed* and not a fellow creature to be nursed into health, so long will these shameful disclosures have to be made. The sick, infirm or mad pauper ceases to be a pauper when so afflicted.'

to Henry Bonham Carter, [?] February 1865

'The sick and the infirm require special constructive arrangements. They are not paupers they are poor in affliction. Society owes them every care for recovery. . . . Sickness is not parochial, it is general and human and should be borne by all. . . . You want hospitals as good as the best civil hospitals and the best nurses you can get. . . . Look at the Assistance Publique in Paris . . . you will do no good without such authority.'

Notes to the Poor Law Board, May 1865 (On the need for a central system for the Poor Law infirmaries to be paid out of a general rate.)

'A. The sick, insane, incurable and children must be dealt with separately in proper institutions and not mixed up in infirmaries and sick wards as at present. The care and government of the sick poor is a thing totally different from the government of paupers. Why do we have hospitals to cure and Workhouse Infirmaries in order not to cure? Taken solely from the point of view of preventing pauperism what a stupid anomaly this is!'

Part of Miss Nightingale's memorandum for Mr Charles Villiers, President of the Poor Law Board, October 1865

'All officers of these Infirmaries & Asylums should be appointed & should be responsible to the central authority which is responsible to Parliament . . .

Hence comes the necessity – necessity as I see it – of consolidating the entire medical relief of the Metropolis under one central management which would know where vacant beds are to be found and so be able to distribute the sick as to use all the Establishment in the most economical way.'

> *to Edwin Chadwick, July 1866*
> *(Miss Nightingale's ABC plan envisaged*
> *all the Poor Law infirmary beds under*
> *one central body independent of the*
> *Guardians; this eventually came to pass*
> *with coming of the London County*
> *Council in 1888. She was also looking to*
> *the day when the sick were treated*
> *equally regardless of economic status.)*

'For I have seen in our English Workhouse Infirmaries neglect, cruelty and malversation such as can scarcely be surpassed in some semi-barbarous countries. And it was there that I felt I must found a School for Nurses for Workhouses etc The opportunity has come to late for me to do Workhouse nursing myself, but so it is well done, we care not how.'

> *to Sir John Lawrence, September 1864*
> *(Sir John's niece, Agnes Jones, was to*
> *pioneer 'Workhouse Nursing' in*
> *Liverpool where she died from typhus*
> *and sheer exhaustion in 1868.)*

'We have been sending our Earls, Archbishops and M.P.s to storm him in his den. . . . Keep the pot boiling.'

> *to Harriet Martineau, May 1866*
> *(Miss Nightingale now identified herself*
> *with the Association for the Improvement*
> *of London Infirmaries, who were*
> *lobbying for reform.)*

'It is a cruel disappointment to me to see the Bill go when I had it in my grasp.'

> *to Mme Mohl, 12 July 1866*
> *(On the fall of the Liberal government in*
> *July 1866, and, with it, the hopes of*
> *reform on the lines laid down by the*
> *reformers. Mr Gathorne Hardy became*
> *President of the Poor Law Board*
> *and drafted his own, less radical,*
> *Bill.)*

'Tell them Barkis is willin' – more than willin' – to give them a piece of her mind.'

> *to Douglas Galton, 31 October 1866*
> *(Miss Nightingale offered to give the*
> *new committee set up by Gathorne*
> *Hardy advice on nursing in workhouse*
> *infirmaries. Galton was on the commit-*
> *tee. 'Barkis is willin' ' is, of course, a*
> *quote from Dickens' 'David*
> *Copperfield'.)*

'Before you decide what to do with the land would it not be better to decide what to do with the Poor Law which is rotten to the heart and wants cutting down.'

> *to William Rathbone, March 1867*

'It is *lèse majesté* to ill use the imbecile woman or the dirty child. Philanthropy is the biggest humbug I know. The principle must be not to punish the hungry for being hungry.'

> *to Mr Nightingale, October 1867*
> *(Miss Nightingale is giving reasons for*
> *declining to join the Association for the*
> *Reform of Workhouses. The Association*
> *wanted reform within the system. Miss*
> *Nightingale thought that the system was*
> *'rotten to the heart' and she wanted a*
> *new system. She was advocating central*
> *control and state medicine for the sick*
> *poor.)*

'The more we go into the matter it is evident that the intent of the Poor Law [The 1867 Act] which is to compel so far as it is possible people to find work for themselves, or others to find work for them, under the penalty of poor rates, is a frightful error. It is applying a money test to a moral wrong. The time appears to be approaching when we will have to adopt *a Moral Poor Law* i.e. a law which will compel people to find work for those who have none, irrespective of any rate . . . It is nonsense talking about there being only a certain amount of work in the community.'

> *to William Rathbone, November 1867*

'What would Jesus have done if he had to work through Pontius Pilate.'

> *Private note, 1868*
> *(On fighting the Prime Minister,*
> *Gladstone, on the subject of pauperism.)*

'SIC TRANSIT *IN* GLORI MUNI without affecting any reform.'

to Henry Bonham Carter, 1871 (not
dated)
(On the new Poor Law Act and the Poor
Law Board.)

Penal Reform

'"The Court feels bound to pass a severe sentence". What does that mean? "The criminal is imprisoned for 18 calendar months". What is that for? Merely to keep him out of mischief for that time? or to deter others by terror? or to reform him? We know that the 2nd of these objects is not ever attained and the 3rd is not even aimed at. Would it not be better to let him out? But no . . . And God feels bound to give sentence "of everlasting chains under darkness". Can He too only punish instead of reform?'

Suggestions for Thought, Vol. 2

Florence Nightingale was writing this when there was a public debate about the need to build new, large prisons as a way of dealing with crime. The solitary cell and incarceration concept was opposed by reformers like Howard and Fry who emphasised rehabilitation. The debate is not new.

'The idea of eternal damnation had its origin amid a society which exercised punishment. As soon as mankind sees that there is no such word, that reformation is the only word, eternal damnation will disappear out of our religion and capital punishment will go out together.'

Suggestions for Thought, Vol. 2

'What has "society" done for us? What is the mission of society? of mankind? To civilise and educate us. What does it do for "fallen women" . . . One would have thought that society, which had done so badly by them in their childhood would now wish to remodel them. Not at all. That is not the question . . . To punish is all that is wanted . . .

What restraint does she put on those men who make them what they are? . . . She throws open her doors to them, vicious as they are and like the beggars, whom she puts in prison, while she praises those who give to them (curious anomaly), so she says to the women "Get out of my path". While to him, without whom the women would not have been vicious, she offers her drawing room and her high-bred daughters.'

Suggestions for Thought, Vol. 2

'We who are moralizing have no distinct impression of what the previous life is of any one who has committed murder . . . Can we doubt that, we had, if we understood the framework of the human spirit – in other words its organisation – if we could trace the various influences affecting a man from his birth to the commission of such a crime [murder] we should perceive when and how the inclination to commit it might have been prevented, the mind opened to better influences?'

Suggestions for Thought, Vol. 1

India

Florence Nightingale never ceased to recommend an improved irrigation system, but the expense deterred the government, which thought building railways was more profitable and would, eventually, bring food to the stricken areas.

'So many authorities are hopelessly at variance as to the facts or the basis of any Gov't duty. (In writing this I am not simply writing as a parrot if *parrots* write – for I have laboured thro' and tried to tabulate immense piles of (so-called) Indian statistics myself.) . . .

Hope deferred makes my heart sick: what must the Indian cultivator's be, – and the famines . . . '

to Lord Salisbury, 15 October 1875
(On the irrigation returns.)

'We do not care for the people of India. This is a heavy indictment: but how else to account for the facts about to be given? Do we even care enough about their daily lives of lingering death from causes we could well remove? We have taken their lands and their rule and their rulers into our charge for State reasons of our own.'

Article in Nineteenth Century, *August 1878*

'The moral is this: that unless you improve the sanitary condition of the Civil population you cannot insure immunity for the soldiers from epidemics.'

to J. Pattison Walker MD, October 1865
(On the report of a cholera outbreak.)

'How curious & instructive that is – & how terrible! It shows that someone must again set hard to work to reform the management & laws of those Jails, like Howard & never leave off till he has done. The contrast between men's and women's health & between the cubic space for each startles even me.'

ibid.
(On receiving a report on the conditions in the Jails in India.)

'*Water*: if we had given them water, we should not now have had to be giving them bread: & not only this but to have seen millions (take all the Famines in this century) perishing for want of it, in spite of all the Governm't has done . . .

It is said that *"Thrift"* is what must save the Indian ryot. This is what the S. of S. [Secretary of State] for India says. We have heard of the horse being made to live (or die) on a straw a day: but I do not think that we ever heard before that the horse ought to exercise "thrift" and save his one straw a day. Yet this is what it appears the country ryot has actually done.

There is little danger of pauperisation that for one who threw himself without need on the Relief measures, ten died in silence almost unknown to our Masters . . .

The common people who find it hard to live when bread is cheap, feel themselves about to die when it becomes dear.'

to Sir Louis Mallet, February 1878

'O that I could do something for India which he saved and for which he lived and died.'

to Sir Harry Verney, 1 July 1879
(On the death of Sir John Lawrence,
Viceroy of India, 1863–9.)

References

[1] Shaw G B (1907) *Major Barbara*. Preface, *The Complete Plays*. London: Odhams Press.
[2] Baly M E (1995) *Nursing and Social Change*, 3rd edn, Chapter 6. London: Routledge.
[3] Baly M E (1986) *Florence Nightingale and the Nursing Legacy*, Chapter 5. London: Routledge.

6

On Hospitals and Hospital Administration

Although she regarded hospitals as an intermediate stage of civilisation, Miss Nightingale was an ardent student of hospital design and administration and had visited many hospitals in Europe. When she returned from the Crimea, improving the design of hospitals was one of her urgent missions. She supported people like Dr Farr and Edwin Chadwick in believing that hospitals should be built on high, dry ground away from centres of dense population. Her favoured layout was that of Lariboisière in Paris, with the pavilion system which allowed the circulation of air through the wards. The plan for the Nightingale ward was laid down in *Notes on Hospitals*, and put into practice in many new buildings. Miss Nightingale's interest in St Thomas's arose because she thought it would be rebuilt in the healthy suburbs, preferably on Blackheath (where the Herbert Hospital was eventually built). She never forgave the governors for resiting it in Westminster on the banks of the polluted Thames.

On the subject of administration she was adamant that the head should be a first-rate businessman. Of course, the treasurer was all important because he had to raise the money for the running of the hospital. She had no time for democratic committees and sub-committees, and was in favour of firm line management and central authority. Interestingly enough, her plan for London virtually came true with the London County Council at the end of the century.

Generally speaking, she thought that doctors were poor administrators and she insisted, rightly, that doctors and nurses were only as effective as the system for the delivery of health care allowed them to be.

Notes on Hospitals is worth re-reading in the light of modern problems, for much of it is timeless. Still we complain that hospitals produce iatrogenic diseases and that patients suffer from something other than on the bed ticket, that hospital kitchens are sources of infection and that, in spite of modern ventilation and central heating, patients complain of being too hot or too cold (not to mention Legionnaire's disease) and that nurses do not seem able (or do not regard it as their responsibility) to remedy the situation. Perhaps most interesting is the emphasis on work study and labour-saving devices. 'Time spent on cleaning what had better not have been there to be cleaned' is a lesson that we have only recently learned, if indeed it has been learned. However, Miss Nightingale's plan for those streamlined and open wards and long corridors was partly to ensure that nurses and other hospital servants were always open to scrutiny, and that there were no stairs or concealed cupboards, which were an invitation to 'sulking or gossiping' – or worse. The new nurse was to be the cynosure of all eyes and a paradigm of moral excellence at all times.

'I have visited all the hospitals in London and Dublin and Edinburgh and many county hospitals, some of the Naval and Military Hospitals in England; all the hospitals in Paris and studied with the Soeurs de Charité, the Institute of the Protestant Deaconesses at Kaiserswerth on the Rhine where I was twice in training as a nurse [sic], the hospitals in Berlin and many others in Germany, at Lyons, Rome, Alexandria, Constantinople, Brussels, also the war hospitals in France and Sardinia.'

Introduction to the evidence to the Royal
Sanitary Commission, 1857
(Miss Nightingale exaggerated her
curriculum vitae somewhat to impress
the Commissioners.)

'To God when he speaks Himself they will listen – not to me – It is the usual fate of those who try to put a little commonsense into their fellow men.'

Private note, 1857
(Lying on her couch preparing evidence
to the Sanitary commission.)

'Hospitals are an intermediate stage of civilization. While devoting my life to hospital work I have come to the conclusion that hospitals are not the best place for the poor sick except for surgical cases.'

to Sir John McNeill, August 1860
(This is a sentiment that Miss
Nightingale repeated time and again.)

'My view you know is that the ultimate destination of all nursing is the nursing of the sick in their own homes . . . I look to the abolition of all hospitals and workhouse infirmaries. But no use to talk about the year 2000.'

to Henry Bonham Carter, June 1867
(Quoted by Brian Abel-Smith to the
World Health Conference 'Health for All
by the Year 2000'.)

On Children's Hospitals

'The causes of the enormous child mortality are perfectly well known: they are chiefly want of cleanliness, want of ventilation, careless dieting and clothing, want of white washing; in one word want of *household* care of health. The remedies are just as well known, and among them is certainly not the establishment of a Child's Hospital.'

Notes on Nursing, 1859

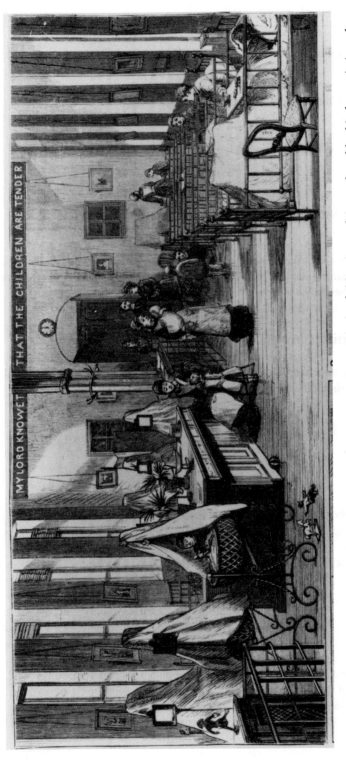

Princess Mary Ward of the East London Hospital for Children in 1878, typical of a children's ward (reproduced by kind permission of the Hulton Picture Company).

'The first thing to decide is whether you will have a children's hospital at all.'

Notes on Hospitals, 1863

'Every sick child may almost be said to require a nurse to herself.'

ibid.

'The true maternal feeling may be found in the girl and in the old maid.'

ibid.

'In all hospitals (and in a children's hospital much more than others) the patient must not stay a day longer than is absolutely necessary.'

ibid.

'There is a tacit idea among some religious [orders] that it is better for children to die than to live. Indeed more tenderness has been shown to them among the commonest hospital nurses.'

ibid.

On Hospitals and Hospital Administration

'It is behind the day. It is not such a hospital as the great Military Hospital of the Empire should be. It would make a model barracks for 2,000 men.'

to John Sutherland, January 1857
(On the design for Netley. Miss
Nightingale tried to persuade Lord
Panmure to change the design, but
failed. Netley was never a success; it
was demolished in 1966.)

'This defies criticism . . . If the object is to build a suitable hospital where people have a chance of recovery – and not to cover a particular piece of ground with buildings – what can one say but only condemn it utterly . . .

And as I don't approve of the principle of Lock Hospitals, I had better let it go on.'

to Douglas Galton, 1861
(On the plans for a Lock Hospital (a
hospital for venereal diseases) in
Devonport.)

'It is impossible to understand on what principles he has placed his W.C. in the middle of the length of one side and his scullery opposite . . .

I am not able to go into the errors of detail in the Offices.

Of all things avoid unnecessary corners in Military Hospitals – additional place to clean (and to skulk in).

The large Hall is an unnecessary expense . . . Military hospitals are to cure the sick; not to be married in.'

> *to Robert Rawlinson, September 1860*
> *(On Dr Combe's paper in* The Builder
> *on his plan for a Regimental Hospital.*
> *Florence Nightingale is defending her*
> *preferred design for the Pavilion.)*

'I would not have sent an angel from Heaven to nurse at Netley in its present state.'

> *to Henry Bonham Carter, June 1869*

'The Hospital books show a considerable proportion of cases are already brought from the purer air of the outskirts. Even if they are brought to St Thomas's they would be better off in a country hospital . . . '

> *Note to* The Builder, *19 March 1859*
> *(Florence Nightingale added her voice*
> *to the campaign to get St Thomas's*
> *rebuilt in the suburbs; she never forgave*
> *them for choosing the present site on the*
> *bank of the Thames.)*

'The position is the worst about London and two feet above the water mark. Dr Leeson's proposal to warm by hot water should not be entertained. Open fireplaces only are permissible.'

> *to R. Baggallay (Treasurer, St*
> *Thomas's), 13 January 1863*
> *(On seeing the plan to rebuild St*
> *Thomas's at the south of Westminster*
> *Bridge.)*

'It may seem a strange principle to enunciate as a first requirement in a hospital that it should do the sick no harm.'

> *Introduction, Notes on Hospitals, 1863*

'Accurate hospital statistics are much more rare than is generally imagined, and at the best they only give the mortality that has taken place in the hospital and take no cognizance of those cases which are discharged in a hopeless condition and die immediately afterwards.'

> *ibid.*

'The patients are suffering from something quite other than the disease on the bed ticket. A vast deal of the suffering and some at least of the mortality in these establishments is avoidable.'

> *ibid.*

'There is a reason for everything.'

ibid.
(On hospital infection.)

'Every five minutes wasted in cleaning what had better have not been there to be cleaned is something taken from and lost by the sick.'

Notes on Hospitals, 1863

'Patients in bed are not peculiarly inclined to catch cold and in England where fuel is cheap, somebody is indeed to blame if the ward cannot be kept warm enough and if patients cannot have bedclothing enough as for as much fresh air to be admitted from without as suffices to keep the ward fresh.'

ibid.

'But the generality of civil hospital kitchens have little to boast of and defective hospital kitchens and bad cooking may be classed as among the causes of hospital unhealthiness.'

ibid.

'From one of our most recently constructed hospitals complaints have been made that there were not sufficient nursing conveniences, that nothing was at hand, that everything had to be sought. Where this is the case the hospital administration must be both inefficient and costly.'

ibid.
(Cf. The Work of Nurses in Hospital
Wards, director J. Goddard, published
1953.)

'Land in towns is too expensive for hospitals. . . . In London the distances are so great and the outward spread of the population so rapid that the question of hospital position assumes quite another aspect from what it does in provincial towns. The problem has been complicated by the nature of hospital foundations which have been created at different periods of time. . . . The practical result has been that several of the largest and most important hospital establishments are concentrated within a comparative narrow area of the metropolitan district. [There follows a map showing twenty hospitals within five miles of St Paul's (reproduced pp. 62–63). Compare this with the Report of Sir Bernard Tomlinson, 1994.]

One result that follows is that a considerable proportion of the sick has been concentrated towards the heart of the metropolis not infrequently among dense masses of population and unhealthy localities. There is no doubt that suburban sites, nearest to the population likely to apply for relief, afford the best solution.'

ibid.

'*Education* might thus take the place of simple instruction.'

ibid.
(On the effect of the above change on
medical education.)

'Sanitary experience has so completely disproved the invisible seminal Contagions that I can only see a mania for being wrong in such letters as Greenhow's & Simon's.'

to Edwin Chadwick, November 1858
(Commenting on letters in The Builder
on the germ theory of infection. John
Simon (later Sir John) became the Chief
Medical Officer to the Central Health
Authority in London and Edward
Greenhow conducted a seminal survey of
sickness in industry; both were pioneers
in Public Health [1].)

'There is no such thing as inevitable infection. Infection acts through the air. Poison the air breathed by individuals and there is infection . . . sick people are more susceptible than healthy people.'

(Notes on Hospitals, 1863)
(In spite of now contrary evidence, Miss
Nightingale is clinging to the miasma
theory, but she is often advocating the
right thing – hospital hygiene – for the
wrong reason.)

'Facts such as these [the high rate of infection and mortality in hospitals] have sometimes raised grave doubts as to the advantages to be derived from hospitals at all and have led many to think that in all probability a poor sufferer would have a much better chance of recovery if treated at home.'

ibid.

'As for doctors civil and military there must be something in the smell of medicine which renders absolute administrative incapacity. And it must be something very strong for they all have an opportunity to develop administrative capacity (almost more than any other profession).'

to Sidney Herbert, 25 May 1859

'The question is purely administrative and good administration is not provided in the Bill [Poor Law Amendment 1867]. What is contemplated is to continue under certain improved conditions the same sort of thing that has existed but with a better system of inspection in the hope that this way evil and neglect will be

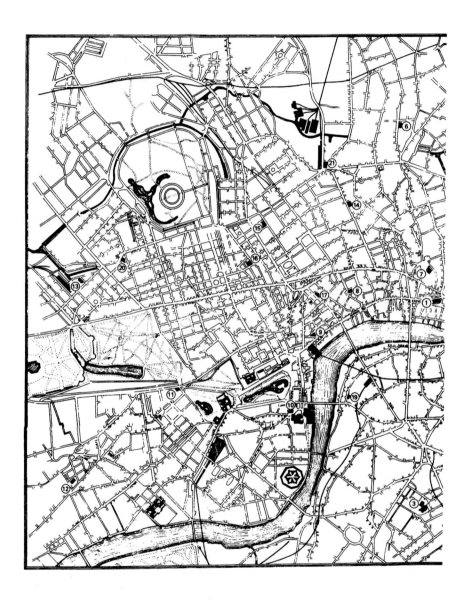

Map of London showing 20 hospitals within 5 miles of St Paul's, pinpointing a problem that is now being resolved (from Florence Nightingale's *Notes on Hospitals*, 1863).

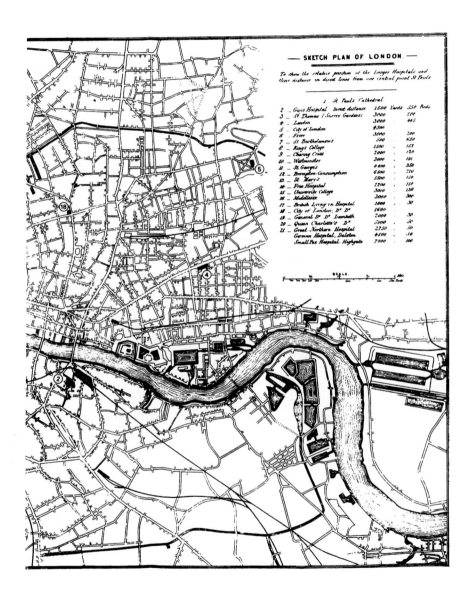

SKETCH PLAN OF LONDON.

To show the relative position of the Larger Hospitals and their distances in direct lines from one central point St Pauls

1	St Pauls Cathedral				
2	Guys Hospital	Direct distance	1500	Yards	550 Rods
3	St Thomas (Surrey Gardens)		3000		200
4	London		4500		445
5	City of London		3000		
6	Fever		3000		200
7	St Bartholomew's		500		650
8	Kings College		1500		152
9	Charing Cross		2000		120
10	Westminster		3000		191
11	St George's		4400		350
12	Brompton Consumption		6500		210
13	St Mary's		5500		150
14	Free Hospital		2200		110
15	University College		3000		138
16	Middlesex		3000		300
17	British Lying in Hospital		1000		30
18	City of London; Do Do		1600		
19	General Do Do Lambeth		2000		30
20	Queen Charlotte's Do		5000		31
21	Great Northern Hospital		2750		50
	German Hospital, Dalston		4500		54
	Small Pox Hospital. Highgate		7000		100

SCALE

prevented. But this is the very principle of administration to be avoided. Inspection involves in it the idea of lax administration and failure to be remedied by punishing somebody for neglect of duty. This is fatal. The real principle should be to provide one *uniform central management* for the whole metropolis and all hospitals should be managed by paid responsible officers under conditions which could easily be framed to ensure success. The head of administration should be a first rate business man . . . '

to J. Parkinson (Poor Law Board),
February 1867

'Doctors are very liable to imagine that because they are the proper people, and only persons to give orders respecting the treatment of patients, therefore they must have the control of the whole staff.'

Henry Bonham Carter to Lord
Beauchamp, August 1872, and repeated
by Miss Nightingale

'What cruel mistakes are sometimes made by benevolent men and women in matters of business about which they know nothing and think they know a great deal.'

Notes on Nursing, 1859

'Hospital were made for patients, not patients for hospitals.'

Hospitals and Patients, 1880

Reference

[1] Baly M E (1995) *Nursing and Social Change*, 3rd edn, p. 100ff. London: Routledge.

7

On Women

Miss Nightingale was strangely contradictory in her attitude to her own sex. No one railed more than she about the limitations society imposed on women and the lack of opportunity for women to engage in worthwhile work. Volume two of *Suggestions for Thought* (much of it lifted from *Cassandra*) is one long diatribe about the wrongs suffered by women in language that at times verges on the hysterical. Virginia Woolf describes her as 'shrieking aloud in her agony' [1]. Florence Nightingale was a campaigner for Women's rights in the first wave of feminism, and in particular women's property rights. This is exemplified by her attitude to the Caroline Norton case in the late 1830s. Caroline Norton's divorce had been a cause celébrè when she, having been abused by her husband, tried to get the custody of her children and the right to her own property, both being denied under English law until 1870.

This period included such women as Elizabeth Barrett Browning, Mrs Gaskell, George Eliot and the radical Harriet Martineau, all of whom Florence Nightingale knew, and others like the Brontës who struggled for recognition in a hostile world. She disagreed with George Eliot when her heroine, Dorothea, in *Middlemarch* married for love, and sacrificed her money and her housing scheme, 'Why could she have not followed the example of Octavia Hill?', asked Florence.

On the other hand she was often very hard on women. When she was young she had 'passions' on female relatives and friends, but that was a common characteristic of the upper class Victorians, probably due to close family ties and the sheltered existence of young women.

In spite of her vitriolic attacks on the family as an institution, Florence Nightingale never ceased to be grateful to her father for the education he had given her. It was the education of an upper class man and she had the intelligence to benefit from it. She was trained as a 'political animal' and except for a few select friends like Mary Clarke, she preferred to work and correspond with men. Her attitude to women was patrician and aristocratic. Conveniently forgetting her own years of struggle, she argued that she had achieved her objectives by giving up all 'for the sake of the work'; any woman could do the same if they had sufficient dedication.

As she grew older she was irritated by what she called 'shouting women' and the clamour of women to enter male preserves like medicine and to have the vote. Bearing in mind her strictures on the Church of England because they did *not* offer women meaningful work, like the Church of Rome, one wonders what her attitude would have been to the ordination of women. Florence Nightingale always maintained that there was plenty of work for women to do in nursing, midwifery and teaching without being 'third rate men'. However she forgot that she had a private income of £500 a year (later increased to £2000) her royalties, a house in Mayfair and five servants and she was later to admit that she had been insensitive to the needs of ordinary women who needed a salary to provide themselves with a reasonable standard of living. Towards the end of her life she softened her views on women in medicine, and her last doctor was a woman. By that time her memory was failing, so perhaps Dr May Thorne's task was less daunting than it might have been.

Florence Nightingale constantly argued that the lack of the vote was the least of women's disabilities. Would it do women any good if they had it? In this history has maddenly proved her right. The economic disabilities suffered were *not* overcome by suffrage; women voted as their husbands and fathers and Victorian male judgement had been internalised by women in a way that enslaved them more profoundly than legal restrictions. The position of women was not fundamentally changed until after the impact of two world wars.

With regard to her family, in bouts of self pity, particularly after the deaths of Sidney Herbert and Arthur Clough, she was excessively hard on, and ungrateful to, her family, who remained remarkably loyal and indulgent. Her public rhetoric is strangely at odds with her private letters to 'Dearest Mum' and 'Pop', and she valued her father's opinion on almost every subject. Far from being abused by her family, she used them ruthlessly (see genealogical tables, pp. 126–127). After 1857 at least four members of the family were actively engaged in the work of the Nightingale Fund Council, not to mention Fanny looking after sick nurses at Embley, Uncle Sam dealing with the accounts and Parthe entertaining the Nightingale nurses at Claydon.

As she grew older, she became an indulgent aunt and spent much time petting and penning sentimental letters to nieces and favourite nurses, which is strangely at odds with the acerbic diatribe against the family as an institution, written when she was young. As far as the nurses were concerned, alas, most of them let her down. They married and 'forsook the work', they supported new fangled ideas like the British Nursing Association, started nursing homes, went abroad or, like the beloved 'Pearl', joined the Church of Rome. Like many elderly ladies, Florence Nightingale did not have a high opinion of modern young women and, like other eminent Victorians, she was inclined to suffer from hubris.

'The maxim of doing things in "odd moments" is a most dangerous one. Would a painter spoil a picture by working at "odd moments"? If it be a picture worth painting at all . . . he must have the whole picture in his head every time he touches it . . . Can we fancy Michael Angelo running up and putting a touch to his Sistine ceiling at "odd moments"?'

Suggestions for Thought, Vol. 2
(from 'Cassandra', 1852)
(In 'Cassandra', Florence Nightingale
developed the theory that women had not

*become 'Beethovens', 'Walter Scotts' or
'Murillos' because they had neither time
nor space to develop their creative
potential, a theme taken up by Virginia
Woolf in A Room of One's Own [1].)*

'Half the people in the world [women] have, indeed no power of thinking . . . But half the world cannot think because they have never tried.'

[There follows a long description of the trivialities that fill a woman's day and why they do not think and write.]

'Few, except Descartes, ever thought without a pen in their hands.'
*Suggestions for Thought, Vol. 2
(On family life.)*

'Women don't consider themselves as human beings at all. There is absolutely no God, no country, no duty to them at all, except family.'
*Private note, [?] 1850
(From 'Butchered to make a Roman
Holiday'.)*

'Jesus Christ raised women above the condition of mere slaves, mere ministers to the passions of man, raised them by His ministry to be ministers of God. He gave them moral activity. But the Age, the World Humanity must give them intellectual cultivation (&) spheres of action.'
'Cassandra', 1852

'The Queen has really behaved like a hero. Has buckled to business at once. . . . She is the only woman in these realms, except perhaps myself [*sic*] Who has a *must* in her life who can set aside private grief to attend res publica.'
*to Mary Mohl Clarke, December 1861
(Florence Nightingale is comparing her
grief on the death of Sidney Herbert and
Arthur Clough with the Queen's grief on
the death of Albert.)*

'Dear Papa,
It would have done me so much good to have had one drop of sympathy, I who for 4 years have never had a word of feeling from my *family* tho' I am sure they have never seen anyone so strained to the utmost pitch of endurance of body and mind as I am. Adieu.'
*to her father, [?] 1861
(On the departure of Aunt Mai, who she
never forgave.)*

Dear Papa,
'Indeed your sympathy is very dear to me . . . '

> *to her father, August 1861.*
> *(On the death of Sidney Herbert.)*

Dear Mother,
So far from being a bore you are the only person who tells me news . . . Thank you so much for the weekly box, tell Burton that I ate a piece of her rabbit pie, which was the first real meat I had eaten for 3 months . . . If you could send me up some snowdrops, primroses, anemones & other wild flowers with roots. I have a fine balcony here looking on Chesterfield Gdns where I mean to take out a licence for rural sports and kill cats . . .

   dear mum
     Your loving child

> *to Fanny, March 1862*

'The real fathers and mothers of the human race are NOT the fathers and mothers according to the flesh. I do not know why it should be so. It "did not ought to be so". But it is. A pretty girl meets a man and they are married. . . . The children come without their consent even being asked because it cannot be helped. . . . For every one of my 18,000 children, for everyone of these poor tiresome Harley Street creatures, I have expended more motherly feeling and action in a week than my mother has expended on me in 37 years.'

> *Private note, 1857*
> *(At this time, there are letters to her*
> *mother thanking her for all her kindness,*
> *for her news and for the parcels of game*
> *and fruit that Fanny always showered on*
> *her daughter.)*

'I have a great horror of being made use of after my death by Women's Missionaries and those kinds of people. I am brutally indifferent to the wrongs or rights of my sex.'

> *to Harriet Martineau, 30 November*
> *1858*

'In the years I have passed in government offices I have never felt the want of a vote, because if I had been a Borough returning two M.P.s I should have had less administrative influence.'

> *to John Stuart Mill, 1863*
> *(For a large part of her active life,*
> *Florence Nightingale had several MP*
> *friends and relatives to ask questions for*
> *her; these included Sir Harry Verney,*
> *Lord Houghton and William Rathbone.)*

'In England, the channels of female labour are few, narrow and overcrowded.'
Subsidiary Notes as to the Introduction
of Female Nursing into Military
Hospitals in Peace and War, 1858

'The greater part of female misery is due to economics, not to the economic position of women specifically, but to the situation of the whole nation, the frightful burden of pauperism. Does Mr Mill really believe that giving any woman the vote will lead to the removal of even the least of these evils?'
to Benjamin Jowett, 1863

'Poverty, not innate depravity, is the cause of prostitution . . . rescue work must include training in gainful skills, caring for silk worms, printing, weaving and farm work which would sustain a girl when she left and equip her for emigration . . . '
to Henry Manning (c Cardinal 1875),
[?] 1852

'Prostitution could not be stopped anymore than I can stop my cat lapping milk . . .

There is no satisfactory evidence that syphilis is propagated *only* by contact with infected persons.'
Note on the supposed Protection
afforded against Venereal Disease by
recognising Prostitution and Placing it
under Police Regulation, 1863

Miss Nightingale gave her name to the campaign against the Contagious Diseases Acts* partly because they suggested the 'germ theory', which was anathema to her, and partly because they implied that the soldier was 'an unmanageable animal' and because the Acts did nothing to look at the problem of the customer.

'If I were to write out of my experience I would begin, *women have no sympathy.* . . . I have never found one woman who has altered her life one iota for me or my opinions. Now look at my experience with men. A statesman past middle age . . . out of sympathy with me remodels his whole life and policy and learns a science, the driest and most technical, that of administration as far as it concerns the lives

---

* The Contagious Diseases Acts 1864, 1866 and 1869 were enacted to check the spread of venereal disease among soldiers and sailors in English and Irish garrison and port towns. The legislation allowed the registration and periodic, compulsory medical examination of prostitutes, who could be held for up to six months if found to be infected. Men were not subjected to the legislation. After a long and bitter campaign, the Acts were repealed by the end of the century.

of men by writing regulations in a London room by my sofa with me. Another, (Alexander whom I made Director General) does very nearly the same thing. He is dead too. Clough, a poet born if there ever was one, takes to nursing administration in the same way for me. I mention only three whose lives were remodelled by sympathy for me. I could mention many others, Farr, McNeill, Tulloch, Storks, Martin and most wonderful of all, Sutherland . . . all these elderly men. Now just look at the degree in which women have sympathy – as far as my experience is concerned . . . No Roman Catholic Supérieure has ever had charge of women of different creeds that I have had. No woman has excited "passions" among women more than I have. Yet I leave no school behind me. My doctrines have taken no hold on women. Not one of my Crimean following has learnt anything from me, or gave herself one moment after she came home to carry out the lessons of war or those hospitals. No woman that I know has ever *appris à apprendre*. And I attribute this to want of sympathy. . . . Women crave for *being loved*, not for loving. They scream at you for sympathy all day long, they are incapable of giving *any* return, for they can't remember your affairs long enough to do so . . .

I am sick with indignation at what wives and mothers will do of the most egregious selfishness. And people call it maternal or conjugal affection, and think it pretty to say so. . . . Ezekeil went running about naked "for a sign". I can't run about naked because it is not the custom of the country. But I would mount three widow's caps on my head "for a sign". And I would cry, This is for Sidney Herbert, This is for Arthur Clough, and This, the biggest widow's cap of all, is for the loss of all sympathy on the part of my dearest and nearest [Aunt Mai, who had gone home to her family].'

to Clarkey (Mme Mohl), 13 December
1861

'I am sorry to say that nurses of ours have been made superintendents who were totally unfit for it and who we earnestly remonstrated with, as well as their employers, to prevent them being made superintendents but in vain – such is the lack of proper persons.'

to Harriet Martineau, 1865
(The argument being that most women
were not fit for responsibility.)

'The more chattering and noise there is about Women's Mission the less of efficient women can be found. It makes me mad to hear people talk about unemployed women. If they are unemployed it is because they won't work.'

to Sir John McNeill, 1865

'No one can be more deeply concerned than I that women should have suffrage. It is so important for a woman to be a "person" but it will be years before you obtain suffrage for women. In the meantime there are evils that press more hardly on women than the want of suffrage. Could not the existing disabilities as to property and influence be swept away by the legislature as it stands at the present? Till a married woman can be in possession of her own property* there can be no love or justice. But there are other evils as I need not tell you. It is possible that if women's suffrage is agitated as a means of removing these evils, the effect may be to prolong their existence.'

to John Stuart Mill, 11 August 1867

'Regulations for women are usually made by men who are incapable of devising suitable regulations for women.'

to Harriet Martineau, [?] 1867
(It should be pointed out that this comment, and others like it, were at odds with Miss Nightingale's own practice. The Nightingale Fund Council never had a woman member in Miss Nightingale's lifetime, though there were eminent women educationalists available. The regulations for nurse training were made by men and largely elderly, medical men.)

'Female M.D.s have taken up the worst part of the male M.D. ship of 50 years ago. The women have made no improvement, they have only tried to be "men" and have succeeded in being only third rate men.'

to John Stuart Mill, 12 September 1860

'She [Elizabeth Garrett] starts on the ground that the *summum bonum* for women is to be able to obtain *the same* Licence or Diploma as for men in medical practice. Now I start from exactly the opposite ground. Medical education is about as bad as it can possibly be. It makes men *prigs.*

It prevents any wise, any practical view of disease & health.

Only a few geniuses rise above it.

It makes a man a prig.

It will make a woman prig-ger . . .

She says – how can we satisfy the Examining Boards? Now – every old fogey, like me, knows that if a man is a genius he can't pass (these "Examining Boards"). What makes a man pass is memory, chique – words – that "Examining Boards" are just so many charlatans . . .

---

* On marriage, all of a woman's property became her husband's. He could dispose of it as he wished; she had no right to it. This was finally redressed by The Married Women's Property Act 1870.

Let women begin with the Profession (Midwifery) which is undoubtedly theirs.'

to Sir Harry Verney, 16 April 1867

'But whether this idea [that women should enter medicine] be right or wrong, shall we not do more harm than good in shutting out women?

Let them try: Once we have "free trade" supply and demand will, will they not, adjust themselves: it will be seen by the simple test of utility, of profit and loss, whether *women* doctors can get *practice* and *deserve practice*.

Fortunately for them they cannot make us legislate that the Public *shall* employ *women* Doctors: any more than we can legislate that the Public shall employ men-Doctors from what we think are the best schools.

Give us free trade: & – *let the Public decide.*'

to Henry Acland, 19 April 1876 (6.30 am)

'Dear Sisters, there is a better thing to be than "medical men", that is medical women [i.e. midwives].'

letter in Notes on Lying-In Institutions, 1871

'I am afraid I have been too much enraged by vociferous ladies talking about things they know nothing at all to think of the rank and file.'

to William Wedderburn, 1896 (Letter asking what the vote would do for ordinary women.)

'She does not want to hear facts; she wants to be enthusiastic.'

Comment on Mrs Josephine Butler's campaign to prevent the reimposition of the Contagious Diseases Act, 1896 (This is an extremely uncharitable comment on one who was anything but 'a shouting lady'. In her old age, Miss Nightingale seems to have changed her mind about these Acts and the fact that they discriminated against women, sometimes in the most brutal fashion.

Reference

Woolf V (1929) *A Room of One's Own*. London: Penguin.

8

The Nature of Nursing

'I use the word Nursing for want of a better,' wrote Miss Nightingale, and she changed her mind many times about what was the proper task of a nurse, and who would make the best nurse. After her Crimean experience, she was convinced that nursing must be secular, but, prompted by Kaiserswerth, she thought that working-class girls, suitably supervised and properly motivated, would make the best nurses and cope best with what she admitted was often servile and repulsive hard work.

Originally, the new style nurses were to be missionaries and moral agents in hospitals, which were often corrupt and lawless places; they were to be the light that shone before men and brought comfort to the sick. At this juncture, Miss Nightingale did not see the nurse as the doctor's assistant or the possessor of medical knowledge. The key to her thinking lies in the letter to Sir Henry Acland, when she says that the less medical knowledge that the matron has the better, as it would hinder her 'sanitary practice'. Miss Nightingale was a sanitarian, and many doctors were not. The nurse's task was to bring hygiene and healthy habits to the hospital and patients alike.

However, the coming of Listerian surgery, asepsis and the germ theory changed the nature of nursing. Doctors were now hygienic and they needed the collaboration of nurses in carrying out treatment and surgery, and nurses did need medical knowledge. Miss Nightingale was ambivalent about this change, as will be seen in her attitude to nursing education. Perhaps, however, she alone of her contemporaries saw nursing as a separate profession and the nurse as an autonomous practitioner, and she was alone in being sorry when nurses became the handmaidens of medicine. Nursing was about prescribing and carrying out total care and putting the patient in the best position for nature to act on, and not merely about carrying on treatment.

Florence Nightingale's ideas on the nature of nursing, especially as contained in *Notes on Nursing*, which were in fact written for guidance on nursing in the home, have often been described as the first 'model' for nursing. However, as shown in Chapter 3, her plan, if there was a plan, had a theological basis; God's law was equated with nature, and nature abetted by the nurse would cure and restore the patient. Secondly, Florence Nightingale's great zeal for sanitation which stood her in good stead in the fight against cholera, typhoid and tuberculosis, would not extirpate every disease. It seems that she remained unaware of the nursing problems of much chronic illness. Her model was a sociological one, though once the doctors took a hand in the training of nurses her acolytes wilfully turned to a biological and medical model. However, as we come to realise, more and more, that the problem of good health largely lies outside the health service, Florence Nightingale's model makes sense. She preached 'Give the nation a clean water supply'; today we are saying 'reduce pollution and educate people in caring for their own health'. Once again nurses are arguing that poverty is still an underlying factor in much ill health, and as Florence Nightingale said so succinctly,

'The causes of the enormous child mortality are perfectly well known . . . the remedies are just as well known and among them is certainly *not* the want of a Child's Hospital.'

Notes on Nursing, Duckworth edition,
1959, p.17.

Today we know all too well that the key to the World Health Organisation's aim at *Health for All* lies not in building hospitals, but in providing sufficient nutrition, shelter, work and a clean environment for all. Perhaps the wheel has come full circle.

Notes on Nursing: What it is and what it is not

'I use the word nursing for want of a better. It has been limited to signify little more than the administration of medicines and the application of poultices. It ought to signify the proper use of fresh air, light, warmth, cleanliness, quiet, and the proper selection and administration of diet – all at the least expense of vital power to the patient.'

Duckworth edition, 1959, p. 15

'Every day sanitary knowledge, or the knowledge of nursing, or in other words, of how to put the constitution in such a state as that it will have no disease, or that it can recover from disease, takes a higher place.'

Preface to Notes on Nursing, 1859

'It has been said and written scores of times that every woman makes a good nurse. I believe on the contrary that the very elements of nursing are all but unknown.'

Duckworth edition, 1959, p. 15

'In these and many other similar diseases the exact value of particular remedies and modes of treatment is by no means ascertained, while there is universal experience as to the extreme importance of nursing in determining the issue of the disease.'

ibid., p. 16

'The same laws of health or of nursing, for they are in reality the same, obtain among the well as among the sick.'

ibid.

'There are five essential points in securing the health of houses:
1 pure air
2 pure water
3 efficient drainage
4 cleanliness
5 light.'

ibid. ('Health of Houses')

'All the results of good nursing as detailed in these Notes may be spoiled or utterly negatived by one defect viz: in petty management, or, in other words, by not knowing how to manage that what you do when you are there, shall be done when you are not there.'

ibid. ('Petty Management')

'Unnecessary noise, or noise that creates expectation in the mind, is that which hurts the patient. Unnecessary noise, then, is the most cruel absence of care which can be inflicted either on sick or well.'

ibid., p. 56

'Never allow a patient to be waked intentionally or accidentally is a *sine qua non* of all good nursing.'

ibid.

'A good nurse can apply hot water bottles to the feet or give nourishment ordered hour by hour without disturbing but rather composing the patient.'

ibid., p. 57

'I have often been surprised at the thoughtlessness (resulting in cruelty quite unintentional) of a friend or a doctor who will hold a long conversation just outside the room or in the passage adjoining the room, [of a patient] who is every moment expecting them to come in, or who has just seen them, and knows they are talking about him.'

ibid.

'All hurry and bustle is peculiarly painful to the sick.'

ibid., p. 61

'A great deal is now written and spoken as to the effect of the mind on the body. Much of it is true. But I wish a little more was thought of the effect of the body on the mind.'

ibid., p. 70

'Home made bread or brown bread is a most important article of diet for many patients. The use of aperients may be entirely superseded by it.'

ibid., p. 77

'It is however certain that there is nothing yet discovered which is a substitute to the English patient for his cup of tea.'

ibid., p. 83

'It is commonly supposed that the nurse is there to spare the patient from making physical exertion for himself – I would rather say that she ought to be there to spare him from taking thought for himself. . . . "Can I do anything for you?" says the thoughtless nurse. . . . The fact is, that the real patient will rather go without almost anything than make the exertion of thinking what the nurse has left undone. And surely it is for her, not for him, to make this exertion.'

ibid, p. 115

'If you do not get the habit of observation one way or another (including taking notes) you had better give up being a nurse, for it is not your calling.'

ibid.

'Yet we are often told that a nurse needs only to be "devoted and obedient". This definition would do just as well for a porter. It might even do for a horse. It would not do for a policeman. Consider how many women there are who have nothing to devote, neither intelligence, nor eyes, nor ears, nor hands. They will sit up all night with the patient it is true, but their attendance is worth nothing to him nor their observations to the doctor.'

ibid., p. 131

'It seems a commonly received idea among men and even among women themselves that it requires nothing but a disappointment in love, the want of an object, a general disgust, or incapacity for other things, to turn a woman into a good nurse. This reminds one of the parish where a stupid old man was set to be schoolmaster because he was "past keeping the pigs".'

ibid., p. 143

'Let no one think that because *sanitary* nursing is the subject of these notes, therefore what may be called the handicraft of nursing is to be undervalued. A patient may be left to bleed to death in a sanitary place. Another who cannot move himself may die of bedsores because the nurse does not know how to change and clean him, while he has every requisite of air, light and quiet. But nursing, as a handicraft, has not been treated here for three reasons

1. that these notes do not pretend to be a manual for nursing any more than cooking for the sick.
2. that the writer, who has herself seen more of what may be called surgical nursing, i.e. practical manual nursing, than perhaps any one in Europe, honestly believes that it is impossible to learn it from any book, and it can only be thoroughly learnt in the wards of a hospital.

3. While thousands die of foul air etc., who have this surgical nursing to perfection, the converse is comparatively rare.'

ibid., p. 140

'It is often thought that medicine is the curative process. It is no such thing. Medicine is the surgery of functions, as surgery proper is that of limbs and organs. Neither can do anything but remove obstructions; nature alone cures. ... And what nursing has to do in either case, is to put the patient in the best position for nature to act on him.'

ibid, p. 142

'In watching disease, both in private houses and in public hospitals, the thing which strikes the experienced observer most forcibly is this, that the symptoms or the sufferings generally considered to be inevitable and incident to the disease are very often not symptoms of the disease at all, but of something quite different – of the want of fresh air, or of light, or of warmth, or of quiet, or of cleanliness, or of punctuality and care in the administration of diet, of each or of all of these.'

ibid.

'Experience teaches me that nursing and medicine must never be mixed up. It spoils both ... '

to Dr Henry Acland, 1869

Nursing Salaries

'The only matron they ever had in India was paid £360 a year (and everything found, as the servants say) The highest salaries women receive at all (Queens and actresses excepted) might be secured by us.'

to Henry Bonham Carter, 1865
(Comparisons are difficult, but by
the end of the century few women
were earning more than £500 a year.
It is not true that Miss Nightingale
advocated low pay or expected nurses
to have a private income. She thought
that a well trained *nurse should be*
well paid.)

'I think all working people ought to be helped in both ways viz. 'Savings Banks' & deferred annuities to obtain an independence ...

All that Mr Gladstone is doing in this line, I think is dictated to the wisest policy ... Suppose every nurse could have a deferred annuity of say £50 at the

age of 55 this would be affluence . . . Would you like to write to Dr Farr for the
pension rates calculated by him.'

to Mary Jones, 1861
(On a pension scheme for the nurses at
Kings College Hospital. Florence
Nightingale did not block pension
schemes for nurses as Professor Smith
has suggested [1].)

Nurses' Food

'I am glad to lay before you what my impressions are:-
want of variety
want of milk
They are tired of cold mutton and would like cold ham and more eggs for
breakfast. They would like at *every* meal especially the little lunch about 10.30
am & at supper sufficient pure milk to be placed on the table.

(This is done at poorer London
Hospitals than ours.)
to John Croft, 1881
(John Croft had taken over from the dis-
graced Richard Whitfield as RMO (she
writes to the RMO, not the matron).)

Nursing Practice

'There is an immense amount of Zinc rubbing but I have not met with a single
observation as to whether there was a danger of bed sores.'

to Mary Crossland (Home Sister), 1881
(Comment on the probationer's diaries.)

Nursing Administration

'I pity the people who have all the organising, all the writing, all the speaking to
do, but never see the patients.'

to Elizabeth Roundell, 1896
(Mrs Roundell was writing a life of
Agnes Jones.)

'The place (Edinburgh) is rough but Miss Barclay takes great pains that the food
and the accommodation be thoroughly healthy. Miss B carries the women with

her in everything. The worst of it is she is killing herself. She shares the Night
Watch twice fortnightly.'

to Mary Jones ('dearest ever dearest
friend), 1873
(Unfortunately Elizabeth Barclay had
taken to opium and alcohol (or had
already been addicted) and was forced
to leave. Miss Nightingale spent much
time battling for her redemption [2].)

To Make Nursing an Art

'The first question [for an art] is not whether a person is "a lady", a person
working for her bread, or a person of the lower middle class. I do not see what
this galimatias about ladies, volunteers etc. has to do with it. Is a lady less of a
lady because she has trained herself to such a point she can command the highest
pay? Is a lady less a lady when she is placed in such a position that she can
support her infirm mother or orphan brothers and sisters? . . . She nobly braces
herself and says I will serve God in his poor sick . . . !' .

to the Editor, Macmillan's Magazine,
April 1867

'Nursing is an art; and if it to be made an art, it requires as exclusive a devotion,
as hard a preparation, as any painter's or sculptor's work. For what is the having
to do with dead canvas or cold marble compared with having to do with the
living body – the temple of God's spirit? It is one of the fine arts; I had almost
said, the finest of the fine arts.'

ibid.

Public Health and District Nursing

'My whole life being a hurry: if one thing was done to the day, it would not be
done at all . . . Nursing was a good apprenticeship.'

to Benjamin Jowett, 1865

'Never think that you have done anything effective in nursing in London until
you nurse, not only the sick poor in workhouses, but those at home.'

Private note, Easter 1867

'District Nursing, so solitary, so without cheer and the stimulus of a big corps
of fellow workers in the bustle of a public hospital, but also without many
of its cares and strains requires what it has with you [the M. & N.N.A.]
constant supervision and inspiration of a genius for nursing and a common

Home. May it spread with such a standard all over London and over the whole land!'

Address to the newly formed
Metropolitan and National Nursing
Association, 1874

'The District Nurse must first nurse. She must be of a yet higher class and of a yet fuller training than a hospital nurse because she has no hospital appliances to hand . . . the doctor has no one but her to report to him. She is his staff of clinical clerks, dressers and nurses.'

On Trained Nursing for the Sick Poor,
1876

'Are District Nurses to be doctors in any sense of the word? Indeed are there any real directions given by the doctor to the District Nurse for care and treatment except in rare cases where the doctor sends for the District Nurse? Has the nurse to run after the doctor? Does he make it possible for her to meet him by appointment at the patient's bedside?'

On Trained Nursing for the Sick Poor,
1881

'Besides nursing the patient she shows them in their own homes how they can call in official sanitary help to make their own poor room healthy, how they can improve appliances, how their home may not be broken up.'

Miss Nightingale's introduction to
William Rathbone's The History of
Nursing in the Homes of the Poor, 1890
(dedicated to Queen Victoria)

'We look upon the District Nurse, if she is to be what she should be, and if we give her the training she should have, as a great civilizer of the poor, training as well as nursing them out of ill health into good health, out of drink into self control, but all without preaching, without patronizing – as friends in sympathy. But let them hold the standard high as nurses.'

to the Duke of Westminster (Chairman of
the Commemoration Fund and the
Metropolitan and National Nursing
Association), 16 December 1896

Health Visiting

'I have been making assiduous enquiries for educated women trained in such a way that they could personally bring their knowledge home to cottagers' wives in a mission of health in rural districts. For this they must be *in touch and in love*, so to speak, with poor rural mothers and girls and show them better things without giving offence.

We have, tho' they be but a sprinkling, in one or two great towns and in London, excellent Town District Nurses, but for obvious reasons they would not be suitable for your proposed work. . . . It hardly seems necessary to contrast sick nursing with this. The needs are quite different. Home Health bringing requires different, but not lower, qualifications and more varied. They require tact and judgement unlimited to prevent the work being regarded as interference and becoming unpopular. They require initiative and real belief in Sanitation and that Life and Death may lie in a grain of dust or drop of water or other such minutiae which are not minutiae but Goliaths and the Health Missioner must be David and slay them.'

to Frederick Verney, Chairman, North
Bucks County Council, 17 October 1891

'It is the first real practical experiment of the kind and it is strange that what I have been thinking of half my life I should have to begin in what to me is a foreign land and not the home of my youth.'

to Mrs Norris (née Rachel Williams),
October 1891
(On the North Bucks scheme.)

'Prizes to cottages for cleanliness are not desirable. The prizes ought to be to handy water supply – to the authorities. The first possibility of rural cleanliness lies in water supply.'

to the Medical Officer of Health, Bucks,
November 18[??]

'This scheme [for Health at Home Nursing] contemplates the training of ladies, so called health missioners, so as to qualify them to give instruction to village mothers in: The sanitary conditions of the person, clothes, bedding and home.

The management of the health of adults, women before and after confinement, infants and children.'

Address prepared for the Chicago
Exhibition, 1893

'I look to the day when there are no nurses to the sick but only nurses to the well.'

ibid.

References

[1] Smith F B (1982) *Florence Nightingale – Reputation and Power*, p. 168. London: Croom Helm.
[2] Baly M E (1986) *Florence Nightingale and the Nursing Legacy*, p. 162, ff. London: Routledge.

9

Nursing Education

When Miss Nightingale returned from the Crimea, she had no clear ideas about training nurses. Nursing was not her priority. Nevertheless, she was pressed to write on the subject, and, in 1858, her *Subsidiary Notes* to the Secretary of State for War are surprisingly detailed for one who 'had no plan'. Miss Nightingale had looked at systems of training all over England and Europe and had come to the conclusion that any new system must be secular and aimed at working-class women 'who normally work in hospitals for a livelihood', with perhaps a sprinkling of educated ladies. Hospitals were thought to have a coarsening effect, and such women were to be *sans reproche*; hence the importance of a secure Nurses' Home with supervision. Nurses were not expected to be the doctors' assistants and accounts of the nursing at St Thomas's in 1860 show that the probationers did little treatment; this was done by medical students.*

But the idea that new style 'trained' recruits would 'leaveneth the whole lump' was soon disabused. Unlettered working-class women did not make trainers of others. After seven years, with the resources of the Nightingale Fund now strained, a wastage rate of over 40 per cent and no superintendent material, it was reluctantly decided to try to recruit 'Special Probationers' – women who were educated and who had leadership potential, some of whom might be persuaded to pay for their board and lodging. The Nightingale Fund needed the money. Selection of such candidates was not always wise and sometimes it caused conflict, but Specials coincided with changes in the use of hospitals and the introduction of Listerian surgery. Now there was a demand for medical lectures. Having dreaded nurses becoming 'medical women', we now find Miss Nightingale bowing to the inevitable and saying that St Thomas's must give more advanced lectures in order to keep up with other schools. To her credit, Miss Nightingale saw, and probably alone saw, the danger of the medical model, but having decided that a nursing school must be attached to an acute general hospital, she was powerless to do anything about it. Nor, if she abandoned St Thomas's, did she know what to put in its place. Probably the new style district nurse and health visitor more nearly fulfilled her idea of what a nurse should be, and in her later years we find her more interested in community care and less interested in hospitals.

By the late 1870s, however, what Miss Nightingale wanted or thought was probably irrelevant; the hospitals had taken over. Training schools with large forces of probationer labour were soon to be *de rigueur* in the hospital world. Miss Nightingale complained bitterly and interminably that 'the probationers were doing

---

*See Rebecca Strong's account of nursing in the Surrey Gardens [1].

half the hospital's work' and 'it could hardly be described as training', but her complaints fell on deaf ears – even on the ears of the nurses themselves.

But nursing was 'fashionable', and we see from Miss Nightingale's 'Addresses' that the new nurses were often conceited; they enjoyed the admiration heaped on them and they perpetuated the system that raised them to such a pinnacle. At the same time, the apprentice system, which had evolved so haphazardly, now ensured that the hard-pressed voluntary hospitals could survive and give a respectable nursing service to their growing middle-class clientele. The fate of the voluntary hospitals was soon to be tied with the unending stream of devoted, biddable probationers supplying cheap labour as the price of training. Thus the pattern of nurse education was set for the next century.

What we call the 'Nightingale system' was not devised by Miss Nightingale and was not a 'system'. It was a pragmatic way of teaching nurses on the job and keeping down costs. No one, and certainly not Miss Nightingale, was sure what was the proper task of the nurse, how she should be trained, or what was the central philosophy; there were no criteria for measuring standards of excellence or how a nurse should be tested and examined. Nursing developed, not by evaluating the nursing needs of the community and developing a strategy to meet those needs, but often by taking on tasks that other workers no longer wanted and by carving out a career structure for nursing superintendents.

The Nightingale reforms did not have the spectacular effects claimed by the early nurse historians, but in history what people think is happening is often as important as what actually happened. While the illiterate probationers at St Thomas's were dying of typhoid or being dismissed by an uncomprehending, untrained Mrs Wardroper, the Nightingale Fund Council was trumpeting the success of the scheme in the press. [.] This produced the illusion that nursing *was* becoming a profession for educated women. In a world where opportunities for such women were few, the trickle of educated women coming into nursing was soon enough to change the public perception about its respectability and act as a grain of mustard seed. For better or worse, the so-called Nightingale system took root.

The Education and Training of Nurses

'I would rather than *establish a religious order open a career highly paid*. My principle has always been that we should give the best training we could to any women of any class, of any sect, paid or unpaid, who had the requisite qualifications moral, intellectual and physical for the vocation of Nurse. Unquestionably the educated will be more likely to rise to the post of Superintendent, but *not* because they are ladies but because they are educated.'

to Dr William Farr, 13 September 1866
(On the subject of Dr Stewart's views
that no lady should work for pay and,
for all classes, nursing must be a
vocation and pay not a consideration.)

'Improving Hospital Nurses
This I propose doing not by founding a Religious Order but by training, system-
atizing and morally improving as far as it may be permitted, that section of the
large class of women supporting themselves by labour who take to hospital
nursing as a livelihood, by inducing, in the long run, some such women to
contemplate usefulness and the service of God in the relief of man . . . and by
incorporating with both these classes a certain proportion of gentlewomen who
may think it fit to adopt this occupation.

The main object I conceive to be, to improve hospitals, by improving hospital
nursing, or by contributing towards the improvement of the class of hospital
nurses whether nurses or head nurses.'

> *'Subsidiary Notes as to the Introduction*
> *of Female Nursing into Military*
> *Hospitals in Peace and War'. Presented*
> *by request to the Secretary of State for*
> *War, 1858*

'As regards ladies, not members of Orders, peculiar difficulties attend their
admission; yet their eventual admixture to a certain extent in the work is an
important feature of it. Obedience, discipline, self-control, work understood as
work, hospital service as implying masters, civil and medical, and a mistress;
what service means and abnegation of self are things not always easy to be learnt,
understood and faithfully acted on by ladies. It seems to me important that ladies
have no separate status but should be merged among the head nurses, by whatever name they are called.'

> *ibid.*

'St John's House possesses great advantages. . . . Not because it includes a
Sisterhood, a system in which I for one humbly but entirely disbelieve, but
because the laborious, servile, anxious, trying drudgery of real hospital work
requires like every duty, if it is to be done aright, the fear and the love of God.'

> *ibid.*

On Nurse Training

'The most important practical lesson that can be given to nurses is to teach them
how to observe – how to observe what symptoms indicate improvement – what
the reverse – which are of importance – which are evidence of neglect and what
kind of neglect.'

> *Notes on Nursing (1859), p. 111*

'If a nurse is learning, she can't be *in the place* of another nurse . . .
Not one Midwife is saved by having Pupil Midwives.
As to St Thomas's:

tho' I have often found fault with them for turning a penny out of us it has not been for employing our Probationers as "extra" Nurses for severe cases – not for employing them to take the place of sick or absent nurses – not even for working a whole ward with our Probationers, as has *not never* been done but for helping themselves, as they frequently have done, to our *un*-certificated nurses (Probationers who have only been with us a few months) to fill *permanently* vacant situations as Nurses and Sisters – at St Thomas's. In such a case, either St Thomas's or the women ought certainly to refund to the N. [Nightingale] Fund.

But we have been obliged to submit. Because it has been a choice of having our own women or a stranger as Head Nurse over our Probationers.'

to Sir Harry Verney, 16 April 1867

The Nightingale Fund

During 1855 to 1856, the grateful nation collected £45,000 (about £1 million in today's money) to be given to Miss Nightingale to provide a means of training nurses and hospital attendants [2]. Miss Nightingale herself was far from enthusiastic about the Fund, which she subsequently regarded as a millstone round her neck. Pleading illness, she often tried to get out of the responsibility for its administration. During the first seven years or so, the administration was largely left to the Trustees, the Council and the day-to-day running to Henry Bonham Carter, Miss Nightingale's lawyer cousin, who served the Fund faithfully from 1861 to 1914, and who himself became a considerable authority on nursing. (Were there worlds enough and time, this book might be extended to include 'As Bonham Carter said . . . '.)

St Thomas's drove a hard bargain with the Fund Council and soon they were using the income from the Fund to subsidise the nursing services. After about 1890 the Fund played a comparatively small role in determining the nurse training pattern or in deciding where nurses went. However, it continued with an advisory role and today it offers post-registration opportunities to nurses from any training school.

The Nightingale School at St Thomas's Hospital

'I have no plan . . . if I had a plan it would be simply to take the poorest and least organised hospital in London and putting myself there see what I could do – not touching the Fund for years until experience had shown how the Fund might best be available.'

to Selina Bracebridge, February 1856
(From the Crimea.)

'I find my health so much impaired that I am consequently so unequal to begin a work which to be properly performed will require great exertion, unceasing attention that I feel it incumbent upon me, and to the contributors, to beg you to communicate to the trustees and the Council my inability to undertake the work.'

to Sidney Herbert, 22 March 1858
(Florence Nightingale tried to avoid the
responsibility for the Nightingale Fund
and starting a nursing school; she tried
writing a 'last letter', but Sidney Herbert
insisted that she must shoulder the
burden.)

'I attribute my success to this
I NEVER GAVE OR TOOK AN EXCUSE.'

Private note, 1859
(Apocryphal sources suggest that this is
what Miss Nightingale said to the
Ambassador in Constantinople in 1854.)

'The public subscribed to the Fund, and hospitals, as far as we know, never subscribed 6d. Yet the Fund has been devoted exclusively to the benefit of hospitals, and almost exclusively to the benefit of St Thomas's, which never gave a farthing . . . '

to Henry Bonham Carter, 1867
(They were jointly considering using the
Fund money to promote district nursing.)

On Nursing and Training at St Thomas's Hospital

'It is not the *best conceivable* way of beginning. But it seems to me the *best possible*. It will be a beginning in a very humble way. But at all events it will not be a beginning with a failure, i.e. the possibility of upsetting a large hospital – for she is a tried matron.'

to Sidney Herbert, 24 May 1859
(St Thomas's had refused to have a
separate superintendent for the training
school and had insisted that their matron
must have control over the
probationers.)

'What grounds have we to trust St Thomas's in the selection of another matron – they are the last persons we should trust – everything is won at the point of a sword.'

to Henry Bonham Carter, 4 January
1866

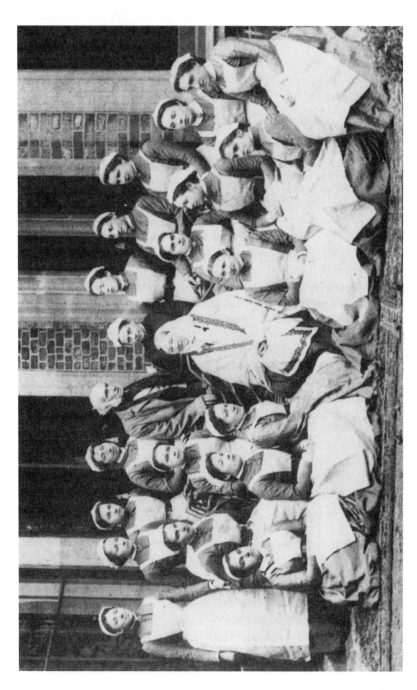

Miss Nightingale with a group of Nightingale nurses from St Thomas's Hospital, with Miss Angelique Pringle as Matron, at Claydon in 1888 (reproduced by kind permission of the Edinburgh Medical Archives).

'We are not dealing with gentlemen.'

> *to Henry Bonham Carter, 1867*
> *(On the officials at St Thomas's*
> *Hospital.)*

'It is easy to potter and cobble about patients for a year without learning the reason for what is done so as to be able to train others.'

> *to Henry Bonham Carter, 1868*

'The chief trainer at St Thomas's was a drinking woman.'

> *to Henry Bonham Carter, 186[?]*
> *(Quoting Mrs Shaw Stewart.)*

'We were the making of St Thomas's they are the unmaking of us.'

> *to Henry Bonham Carter, 1872*

'Our pros do very hard work together with sisters too inexperienced or too dispirited or too driven to care how to make nurses do their proper share so that the probationers shall have what we promise them – a year's training.'

> *to Henry Bonham Carter, 1872*

'you put very ill-educated women under exactly the same circumstances of training as educated women (what are called ladies) – you give them the temptation of boasting of sacrifices which they don't make. And no opportunity is supplied them of knowing or correcting their ignorance – not even their bad spelling.'

> *to Henry Bonham Carter, 1871*
> *(Quoting Miss Torrance (the Home*
> *Sister) who highlighted the problems*
> *facing the School at St Thomas's. Miss*
> *Torrance is drawing attention to the*
> *problem that was to beset nursing for*
> *years to come, that of a wide span of*
> *educational ability in the intake of*
> *probationers/students.)*

1872

Thanks to the introduction from about 1867 of Special Probationers who were better educated and articulate, Miss Nightingale and Henry Bonham Carter began to hear of the deficiencies of the training scheme and the fact that Mrs Wardroper seemed unable to cope with her dual role. At the same time it was discovered that Mr Whitfield, the Resident Medical Officer, was not giving the lectures to the probationers as he was paid by the Fund to do. The Red Register (the character sheet devised by Miss Nightingale) was as 'capricious as if a cat had made it'.

The crisis came in 1872 when the Fund Council took legal advice about the possibility of using the capital and starting again. In the end there was a compromise, which included the enforced resignation of Mr Whitfield as a lecturer, the introduction of a Home Sister as 'Mistress of the Probationers', Miss Nightingale's inspection of the Red Register and regular interviews with the probationers, her addresses to the probationers, and the use of Fund money to start Schools and projects (including district nursing) elsewhere. The quotes that follow largely stem from these facts.

'It has been a universal and increasing complaint among our good probationers that our sisters do not give instructions as promised in the regulations.'

> *to Henry Bonham Carter, 1871*
> *(This complaint is repeated time and*
> *again.)*

'The stupid ones read and are puffed up and don't understand, and they don't know that they don't understand. The clever ones understand enough to know that they don't understand and are discouraged having no one to answer their questions.

I think misguided and purposeless reading the most dangerous of all.'

> *to Henry Bonham Carter on Mr John*
> *Croft's reading list, 1872*

'We are just in time to prevent Mrs W from degenerating into governing like a virago. By talk, by being heard not felt. By speaking more than she observes all of which are the first elements of authority. She maintains authority by self assertion and she is losing it every day . . .

She said, "I can dismiss Miss Cameron and every woman in this place without referring to anyone". This is true, but what a way to enforce authority . . .

Mr Whitfield has been for years in habits of intoxication. For years he has been in the habit of making his rounds at night (at a later hour than anything could justify . . .) oftener tipsy than sober . . . For the past 4 or 5 years Mr W. has done nothing for the probationers, except to exploit his position to the verge (and beyond) of impropriety. I am convinced that "nothing" is literally accurate.'

> *to Henry Bonham Carter, 12 May 1872*
> *(Part of a very long letter in several*
> *parts.)*

'If you could see her [Mrs Wardroper] as I see her because I cannot take up my hat I am sure you would think her brain might go any day.'

> *to Henry Bonham Carter, June 1872*

'Mrs W did not arrange the work or even Bible classes. Nurses left their patients and stood to attention.'

> *to Henry Bonham Carter, 29 November*
> *1872*

'Intolerable conceit is one of our nurses' chief defects.'

to Henry Bonham Carter, 1872
(This was repeated on a number of
occasions.)

'We exact a quantity of menial work from those to whom we hold out a career of training others and superintendence, wholly unnecessary except for the purpose of hospital economy.'

to Henry Bonham Carter, 1873

'If we had experienced sisters, if we had a matron with any system, if we had a head to the Home most certainly with 33–35 pros to 330 patients at least 2 hours a day, besides proper rest and exercise, could be spared for each pro for classes.'

to Henry Bonham Carter, 1873

'There is no training for those who are to train others. Probationers have no means to qualify themselves for superintendence which is what we ourselves held out for them.'

to Henry Bonham Carter, February
1873

'If your Committee [the Nightingale Fund Council] did not pay the pro's board the hospitals would still be the gainer. Really I think under the present circumstances to spend the most we can away from St Thomas's would be most for our school's interest.'

to Henry Bonham Carter, 1873

'The present ward training of our probationers is in dirt, in negligence and gross carelessness . . . even the typhoid patients are not washed.'

to Henry Bonham Carter, 1876

'As we are I am not sure that the hard drive of the pros is a bad thing. At least it knocks the ministering angel nonsense out of them and makes them look on nursing as the urgent businesslike work it really is. But then it knocks something else too out of their heads, to wit goodness and all high aspiration.'

to Henry Bonham Carter, 17 January
1877

'Mr Croft's lectures are excellent but are of the most elementary nature and strictly for nurses. We shall have our Lady P's going elsewhere to get knowledge for there is scarcely a good school that does not give them more than we do.'

to Henry Bonham Carter, 23 March
1879

'The first year of training in the Home is all important for it is there that order and discipline and method (of which possibly the probationers have had nothing as yet in their lives) must be taught or they will not be amenable to ward discipline.'

Note to Henry Bonham Carter during
the Anti-Registration debate of the Select
Committee to the Privy Council, 1892

Comments on Probationers' Reports
(The Red Register)

Miss Nightingale devised a character sheet with fourteen heads to be used by Mrs Wardroper. Each entry was to be marked excellent, good, moderate or imperfect by the Sister in Charge (it was, in fact, like modern market research). When she discovered that the entries were meaningless, Miss Nightingale started seeing the probationers themselves and comparing her assessments with those already in the Register. She wrote her own comments, which often disagreed with those of Mrs Wardroper, in the Register itself. Miss Nightingale's comments are interesting because they show the qualities for which she was looking in nurses; they also show perspicacity and a human side. History does not relate what Mrs Wardroper thought of these comments, if indeed she heeded them; nor do we know if Miss Nightingale's judgement was sound, except by checking, where possible, what happened to the probationers later.

The fact that Miss Nightingale was seeing the probationers, questioning them, checking their diaries and getting reports from her favourite 'Specials' must have caused a certain amount of schism in the nursing services, particularly between the ordinary nurse at St Thomas's and the Nightingale probationers. It is perhaps small wonder that Henry Bonham Carter had, at times, to exercise his considerable diplomatic talents.

'Cororan, Anne
Deficient in both management and steadiness, a coarse, low sort of woman but with capabilities which, had she had a stricter probation would have been a more successful nurse and a better woman. She wanted a good sister over her. Given to the gab and quite untrustworthy.'

'Papps, Anne
This is a flaming character. What, all "goods" tho' only a fair nurse comes out of them all? Truly religious, affectionate, conscientious but excitable and unstable. Has improved at Edinburgh.'

'Horney, Mary (a Special)
Of the highest purpose; of true missionary principles. An awkward body and somewhat so in mind. Rarely meet with one so above every mean pursuit.'

'*Ford, Elizabeth*
Ford's bedmaking was intolerable. . . . In spite of defects this is a very superior woman and under strict supervision may yet do well. She was led away by a bad example. She did what she saw others do and was led by her inferiors. Is penitent and grateful being taken on at Highgate. . . . She was lost for not being under a good sister.'

(Ford made good at Highgate.)

'*Leslie, Sophie*
Miss Leslie has the same amount of "goods" as No. 30 & 32 who narrowly escaped dismissal. Deeply religious, with high principles and strong common sense; full of purpose. Felt the deficiency of her training.'

'*Yarnley, Mary*
A clever woman but of a vulgar mind, capable of control: somewhat inclined to hobnobbing where she likes and spitefulness where she does not. Too much on the level of the nurses she has to superintend.'

(Miss Yarnley died of typhoid as a night nurse at St Thomas's Hospital.)

'*Pyne, Lilian*
Felt her want of ward training. A progressive sort of mind. V. clever but a certain want of balance, rather absorbed in her own mental and spiritual difficulties.'

(Miss Pyne became the successful matron of the Westminster in 1880.)

'*Sparks, Ellen*
A very moderate woman indeed moderate in principles [and] steadiness. Not to be trusted in a general hospital for her own sake; light in her conduct with men. Not moderate in flippancy or impropriety.'

(Miss Sparks later married.)

Miss Nightingale's Comments on the Probationers' Diaries

The probationers, particularly the Specials, were supposed to keep diaries of their ward work. Those that are extant are interesting in showing how the probationers spent their long day. Miss Nightingale now inspected these when they were available. Below are some of the comments she sent to Henry Bonham Carter.

'1   These are the horaries, not of probationers, but ward assistants.
2   We do not glean from these at all what they are doing in their special position of learning or what is being done in the way of teaching.
3   Sister scarcely appears at all and in none as a teacher and trainer.
4   The diaries are interesting as giving some account of menial and dressing

work but they offer not the slightest clue to what the place is doing as a training school.

5   It is impossible to do justice to the probationers without an extra nurse. The sisters must do most of the critical cases themselves – they can only give the probationers the light cases and the menial work because they cannot over-look them because they have no time.

6   The pinning up of checks [counterpanes] takes a ridiculous time.

7   In my opinion it can hardly be called training.'

27 December 1876

Miss Nightingale's Addresses to the Probationers at the Nightingale Schools

Extracts from Miss Nightingale's Addresses are included not because they are examples of wit and wisdom, but rather as an unwitting testimony to the class consciousness and the concerns of the times and as an indication of the social milieu against which nurse training was promoted. With their heavy preaching and exhortations to humility and obedience, they are also a testimony to the fact that a life of isolation, communicating only with her peers on a one-to-one basis, meant that Miss Nightingale was largely out of touch with ordinary young women in the 1880s.

The Addresses were started in 1872 when it was realised that there was little training at St Thomas's and that the remarks in the Red Register 'were as capricious as if a cat had made them'. They were written by Miss Nightingale herself and read out to assembled probationers by a member of the Nightingale Fund Council – usually an elderly gentleman. After Miss Nightingale's death, her niece collected the Addresses and in 1914 published a selection.

This selection is interesting to the nurse historian because the annual exhortation frequently reflects the nursing concern of the moment. For example, the problem of introducing 'Specials' or lady probationers into nurse training – an officer class into a single training – was causing trouble. Then there was the dilemma of doctors' lectures, testing by examinations and the dreaded spectre of state examinations as opposed to character assessment. Again, at a time when Miss Nightingale was criticising the overweening authority of the matron, she is at pains to uphold her authority. The much-quoted maxim about Associations stems from the conflict with the British Nurses' Association. Sentimental sermonising these Addresses may be, but packed in there was often a Nightingale political punch. Miss Nightingale was trying to ensure that the Nightingales did not follow false prophets.

The Addresses are also interesting in that again they show the inconsistency of Miss Nightingale's public utterances and her private opinions. She urges Christian humility and blind obedience to a system of nurse training of which she was profoundly critical and which she found flawed. With few exceptions, her acolytes and the future superintendents took this message of obedience to heart, and this was the tragedy. Future schools were replicas of the early Nightingale school, with theory divorced from practice, the training unplanned and the probationers the main work force of the hospital. St Thomas's did not have a Sister Tutor until 1913.

Nevertheless, these exhortations are worth reading if only because they nail the myth that the Nightingale nurses were educated and beyond reproach. Rosalind Nash, Miss Nightingale's niece, justifying the style, points out that they were written for nurses 'who could barely read and write'. The fact that some Nightingales became leaders and superintendents in spite of the system should not blind us to the fact that the run-of-the-mill nurses often had a limited education.

'They [the ordinary nurses] are placed here, and perhaps only here, on a feeling of equality with educated gentlewomen. Do they show appreciation by thinking we are as good as they? Or by obedience and respect and trying to profit by the superior education of gentlewomen?

1872
(In the same passage, Miss Nightingale
goes on to suggest that the ordinary
nurses can save the ladies from the
harder work.)

'For us who Nurse, our Nursing is a thing, which, unless we are making *progress* every year, every month, every week, take my word for it we are going back.'

1872

'Conceit and Nursing cannot exist in the same person, any more than new patches on an old garment.'

1872

'The first element in having control over others, is, of course, to have control over oneself.'

1872

'You will have to work hard if you wish St Thomas's Training School to hold its own with other Schools rising up.'

1873

'May I pay ourselves even the least little compliment, as to our being less conceited than last year? ... But unfortunately is not our name "up" and "abroad" for conceit? And has it not even been said (tell it not in Gath) "and these conceited Nightingale women scarcely know how to read and write"?'

1873

'Do we look enough into the importance of giving ourselves thoroughly to study in the hours of study, of keeping careful Notes of Lectures, of keeping notes of all types of cases . . . so as to improve our powers of observation all essential if we are in the future to have charge.'

1874

'Is there a great deal of canvassing and misinterpreting of the Sisters and Matron and other authorities? every little saying of theirs? talking among one another about superiors (and finding we were wrong when we came to know them better).'

1874

'You cannot help being missionaries. . . . There are missionaries for evil as well as good.'

1874

'A woman who takes a sentimental view of nursing (which she calls "ministering" as if she were an angel) is, of course, worse than useless. A woman possessed with the idea she is making a sacrifice will never do, and a woman who thinks any kind of nursing work "beneath a nurse" will simply be in the way (And I tell you again, what I have had to tell you before, that we have a great name in the world for conceit).'

1875

'To be a Nurse *is* to be a Nurse: not to be a Nurse only when we are put to the work we like. . . . If we can do the work we don't like from a higher motive till we do like it, that is the test of being a real Nurse.'

1876

'Quietness in dress, especially being consistent in this matter when off duty and going out. And oh! let the Lady Probationers realise how important their example is in these things so little and so great. If you are Nurses, Nurses ought not to be dressy, whether in or out of uniform. Do remember that Christ holds up the wild flowers as our example in dress . . .

Oh my dear nurses don't let people say of you that you are like "Girls of the Period", let them say you are like "field flowers" and welcome.'

1876

'The Nightingale Nurses in a novel it [a medical journal] said would be "an active, useful, clever Nurse". These are the parts I approve of. But what else do you think? "A lively, rather pert and very conceited young woman." Ah, there is the rub. You see what our name is "up" for in the world. This is what a friendly critic says of us, and we may be sure that unfriendly critics say much worse.'

1876

To Night Nurses

'Keep to regular hours for your meals, your sleep, your exercise. If you do not you will never be able to stand up to night work perfectly; if you do there is no reason why night nursing may not be as healthy as day (I used to be very fond of the night when I was a Night Nurse: I know what it is. But then I had my day work to do besides; you have not).'

1879

'What makes us endure to the end? Discipline. Do you think that these men could have fought at a desperate post through the livelong night [the 120 men defending a hospital against the Zulus] if they had not been trained in obedience to orders and acting as a corps, yet each man doing his own duty rather than every man going his own way . . . '

1879

'And what is it to obey? To obey means to do what we are told and do it at once. With the nurse, as with soldiers, whether we have been accustomed to it or not, whether we think it right or not is not the question. Prompt obedience is the question. We are not in control but under control . . . we come into the work to do the work . . . '

1879

In the Addresses, Miss Nightingale was very fond of the analogy between the nurse and the private soldier, but twenty years earlier (in *Notes on Nursing*) she had firmly refuted the idea that 'to be devoted and obedient' was enough for a nurse.

'There is no magic in the word Association. . . . We must never forget that the "individual" makes the Association. What the Association is depends on its members. A Nurses' Association can never be a substitute for the individual nurse. It is she who must, each in her own measure, give life to the Association, while the Association helps her.'

1888

What Makes a Good Training School?

'Training is to teach not only what is to be done, but how to do it. The physician or surgeon orders what is to be done. Training has to teach the nurse how to do it to his orders and to teach, not only how to do it, but *why* such a thing is done and not such and such another; also to teach symptoms, and what symptoms indicate, of what disease or change and the "reason why" of such symptoms.

'Nurses Training of, and Nursing the Sick', 1882
(Published in Sir Robert Quain MD, A Dictionary of Medicine.)

'At least a year's practical and technical training in hospital wards under *trained* head nurses who themselves have *been trained to train.*

A second year, if possible, as a ward nurse, day and night, with the benefit of further theoretical instruction.

For a district nurse at least an additional 3 months training of nursing the poor (at home) under a trained and training district superintendent is essential.'

ibid.

'The training of probationers should be as much part of the duty of the head nurse [sister] as directing under nurses or as seeing to the patients.'

ibid.

Records

'Weekly records under printed heads corresponding with the list of duties kept by the head nurses of the progress of each probationer in her ward work and moral qualities. A monthly record by the matron of the results of the weekly records and a quarterly statement by her as to how each head nurse has performed her duty to each probationer.'

ibid.

Lectures

'Clinical lectures from hospital professors; lectures on subjects connected with the nurses' special duties such as elementary instruction in chemistry, with reference to air, water, food, etc. Physiology with reference to the leading functions of the body. General instruction on medical and surgical topics, with examinations, written and oral, at least four times a year. . . . Also lectures with demonstrations with anatomical, chemical and other illustrations – all in the presence of the Lady Superintendent and mistress of probationers [Home Sister] . . . '

A good Nurses' Library of professional books, not for probationers to skip and dip at random, but to be made careful use of under the medical instructor and the class mistress.

Classes for a competent mistress to drill the professional teaching into the probationers' minds. The Mistress of the Probationers to be above all a Home Sister capable of making the home a real *home* and of training and disciplining the probationers there in all good, moral qualities, customs, habits and manners without which no woman can be a nurse . . . '

ibid.

'The authority and discipline over all women of a trained Lady Superintendent who is also the matron of the hospital, who is herself the best nurse in the hospital . . . '

ibid.

'Accommodation for sleeping, classes and meals; arrangements for time and teaching work, surroundings of a moral and religious, hard working and sober yet cheerful tone and atmosphere such as to make the training school and hospital a home which no good young woman of any class need fear by entering to lose anything of health of body or of mind; with moral and spiritual help and an elevating and motherly influence overall . . .

Let nurses be proud of their alma mater. Let there be friendly rivalry with other hospitals and never try to fuse nurses into one mass – one indistinguishable mass – of all training schools or hospitals.'

ibid.

On Marriage

'They had much better see nothing of any Doctors, consulting or Residential except in Hospital. One does not want them to be on visiting terms with Doctors.'

to Mary Crossland (Home Sister), 1896
(Miss Nightingale regarded nurses who
married as' Forsaking the Work'. She
seldom kept up with those who did.)

On Badges and Certificates

'Are we not a bit young for the Garter?'

to Henry Bonham Carter, [?] 1887
(On the suggestion that certain nurses be
given the Order of St Katherine.)

'I cannot help regretting the present rage for certificates and badges. The certificate does to make the nurse, nor does the badge distinguish her as to excellence. Some of our best nurses are without either.'

to William Rathbone, March 1900

Community Nursing

'The object of the whole course being the new one not simply to give Sanitary information but to teach how to teach – the examination by an independent well-known Sanitary authority – both in writing and by word of mouth (to test their power of speaking to the uneducated) . . .

Just as the District Nurse goes into the cottage to nurse and to teach the Patient – the object lesson of the latter being the Cottager's home and its inmates – the rural domestic life – so would the Health Nurse [Missioner] teach what to do in the cottage for health with her own head & hands . . .

Of course it will take a *long* time before prejudice & ignorance are over-come.

to George H. De'ath, Esq., MD, 29 May
1892
(On Health Missioners' Course in
Buckinghamshire.)

References

[1] Baly M E (1986) *Florence Nightingale and the Nursing Legacy*, pp. 54–55. London: Croom Helm/Routledge.
[2] Baly M E (1986) ibid., p.17.

10

The Management of Nursing

Miss Nightingale's experience in the Crimea had clearly demonstrated that the organisation of nursing services was as important as direct nursing care itself. She had clear ideas not only on how hospitals should be organised but also of the nurses' role in such management. In *Notes on Nursing* (1859) she included a whole chapter on petty management. The pronouncement by Sir Roy Griffiths, that 'if Miss Nightingale were alive today she would be looking round to see who was in charge' is a total misunderstanding. Miss Nightingale would have been in charge.

As Miss Nightingale was to say time and again, the whole reform of nursing was about making the matron supreme in nursing matters. 'Don't let the doctor make himself the head nurse and there is no worse Matron than the Chaplain.' 'Woe unto the man who comes between the matron and her nurses.' No one was to have charge of nurses who had not herself been through the training as a nurse.

It is perhaps worth recalling Henry Bonham Carter's repartee during the registration debate, when doctors and administrators had put up an argument for being in charge of nurses: 'When these gentlemen had had control they had not made a very good job of it.'

The idea of 'superintendence' held out a much-needed career structure for nurses and was frequently quoted as an inducement to entering nursing. When the Senior Nursing Structure was introduced (1967), it was not, as some suggested, contrary to the Nightingale system; trained nurses were always in charge of the nursing staff.

Therefore the Nightingale system of nurse training was not only about training nurses to give good bedside care, but also about producing hospital matrons, or, as Miss Nightingale called them, 'trainers of nurses'. In vain Miss Nightingale and Henry Bonham Carter struggled to provide a special course for those pupils intended for superintendence, Mrs Wardroper and St Thomas's always found reasons why not. However, in Edinburgh, Miss Pringle was more co-operative, and those who were considered superintendent material were encouraged and coached. Although Miss Nightingale is usually credited as being the 'Founder of Modern Nursing' a more correct title would be 'a Founder of Modern Nursing'. During the nineteenth century, both in England and in Europe, there were a number of well educated, upper class women looking for a vocation and worthwhile work and, as John Stuart Mill said, 'Occupations, law & usage made accessible to them are comparatively few' and a number looked to nursing; later in the century they might well have turned to medicine. In order to provide themselves with training they sometimes paid for instruction with medical men. Richard Whitfield supplemented his income in this way. But besides paying for tuition at home, many went abroad to the hospitals of Europe and to that Mecca of Protestant social reformers, Kaiserswerth. Miss

Nightingale herself was eclectic and she picked the brains of women like Jane Shaw-Stewart, the superintendent in Crimea, Lucy Osburn, who had nursed all over Europe, and Mary Jones of the Order of St John's at King's College, who gave advice on the programme at St Thomas's and was constantly consulted; this is not to mention all she learned from Mother Clare Moore. The training and administration that eventually emerged at the Nightingale School was the result of much letter writing and consultation with these ladies, who have not been sufficiently acknowledged by posterity.

An aspect of Miss Nightingale's precepts for administration that would appeal to today's hospital accountants was her requirement that change should be cost-effective. Was gas going to be cheaper than a candle allowance to Sisters? Another Nightingale tenet that has a modern ring was the insistence on labour-saving devices or materials. Down to methods of 'blacking' grates, no consideration was too trivial for her exhortation and advice.

In spite of no formal training, educated women with leadership material did go forth and set up other training schools, thus spreading a version of the Nightingale system.

On the Supremacy of the Matron

'The whole reform of nursing both at home and abroad has consisted of this. To take all power out of the hands of men and put it into one female trained head and make her responsible for everything regarding the internal management and discipline being carried out. Don't let the Doctor make himself the Head Nurse and there is no worse Matron than the Chaplain.'

to Mary Jones, Superintendent of St
John's nurses at University College
Hospital, 1867

'My views are exceedingly altered as to the supremacy of the matron. It did very well for me whose fault is subserviency and civility. It does very ill for matrons whose fault is the love of power and lawlessness towards medical and other authorities, and for matronship where there is not the strong and intelligent administration with the power and duties running parallel to the matrons.'

to Henry Bonham Carter, April 1878
(In the late 1870s, there had been a
number of disputes between the new
style matrons and the hospital
administrators.)

'All the results of good nursing as detailed in these Notes may be spoiled or utterly negatived by one defect viz: in petty management, or, in other words, by not knowing how to manage that what you do when you are there, shall be done when you are not there.'

Notes on Nursing (Petty Management)
1859

'How few men, or even women, understand either in great or in little things what it is the being "in charge" – I mean how to carry out a "charge". From the most colossal calamities down to the most trifling accidents, results are often traced (or rather *not* traced) to such want of someone "in charge" or of his knowing how to be "in charge".'

ibid.

'It is often said that there are few good servants now: I say there are few good mistresses now.'

ibid.

'People who are in charge often seem to have a pride in feeling that they will be "missed", that no-one can understand or carry on their arrangements, their systems, books, accounts etc but themselves. It seems to me that the pride is rather in carrying on a system, in keeping stores, closets, books, accounts etc, so that anybody can understand and carry them on.'

ibid.

'The everyday management of a large ward, let alone of a hospital – the knowing what are the laws of life and death for men, and what the laws of health for wards – (and wards are healthy or unhealthy, mainly according to the knowledge or ignorance of the nurse) – are not these matters of sufficient importance and difficulty to require learning by experience and careful enquiry, just as much as any other art.'

ibid. (Conclusion)

Visitors [to Nurses]

'These women are apt to feel and say "we are not in a nunnery" nor should they be. Still on the whole considering the nuisance of ordinary visitors and the greater nuisance of the extraordinary I think if it were possible to make a rule that no visitors are allowed it would be a great gain. I am not sure whether it is possible or not, or still less whether it is possible to keep such a rule . . . '

Subsidiary Notes, 1858
(Subsidiary Notes were written for the
War Office and were the result of Miss
Nightingale's experience in the chaos
and brutality of military hospitals where
it was important to keep female nurses
above suspicion. If the experiment was
to succeed the nurse must be, and be
seen to be, sans reproche.)

Night Nurses

'The night nurse should be on duty 12 hours with instant dismissal if found asleep and 4 hours for daily exercise or private occupation. . . . I would not, however, prohibit occupation at night as sometimes ward duty is slight. . . . I do not fancy, but at present am not positive about, cleaning or scrubbing at night.'

ibid.

Holidays

'Holidays should be distributed in rotation during a fixed time of the year and comprehended in 2 or 3 months or 4 at the outside.'

ibid.

Hospital Economy

'Some years ago gas was laid on in the Sisters' rooms in Guy's hospital. In other hospitals there is an allowance of candle to each sister. The disadvantages of gas are its alleged unhealthiness and its uncertainty being disagreeable to some eyes. Its advantage is its cheapness. Liberty to buy a candle and not use gas is allowed at Guy's. As it will be a very important thing to conduct the nursing service as cheaply as possible, and as there must not be any wretched false economy as to essential matters, which in the end always proves waste it will be well to save as much as can be in matters not essential. It would be worthwhile to ascertain the average amount of saving which the substitution of gas for an allowance of candle has effected at Guy's.'

ibid.

Grading of Nurses

'Guy's had the same provision with, however, the drawback that there was not a Sister in charge, but a nurse over other nurses with higher pay, but not a Sister or Head Nurse. However excellent such a Nurse may be every ward *must* be under some regular government as is general in the hospital if discipline and order are not to suffer.'

ibid.

Military Nurses

'But it may be clearly enunciated what the duties of Female Nurses should be and there will never be discipline in military hospitals until they are as follows:
    Women only of character, efficiency and responsibility. They should have charge and be responsible for all that pertains to the bed-side of the patient; for his cleanliness and that of his bedlinen and utensils, for all the minor dressings

not performed by Surgeons or Dressers, for administration of medicines and of meals, for the obedience of the patient and orderlies to the orders of the M.O. They should receive the orders of the latter and always attend his visits.

Till the above is done by women the same want of discipline, now to be observed in Military Hospitals, and often already noticed will continue – such is my firm belief, the result of much experience.'

ibid.

Comparison with Civil Hospitals

'All the patients are men . . . There are nurses under a matron and orderlies under some officers and there is no civil element. Doctors both prescribe and hitherto have governed. An officer orders flogging etc. but Doctors practically have governed. A Military Hospital must, and should ever remain, essentially different from a Civil Hospital, both different in discipline and detail and altogether a rougher and ruder place.

Discipline then being the pivot upon which the good order of all Military things, Military Hospitals included, it follows that if you set down a few women in a great Military Hospital, unless they become effectually incorporated into the general spirit of discipline of the place they will injure themselves and the whole.'

ibid.

Nurses in Civil Hospitals

'The head nurse should be within reach and view of her ward both day and night. Associating nurses in large dormitories tends to corrupt the good and make the bad worse. Small airy rooms contiguous to the wards are best. The wards should have one entrance and the head nurse's room should be close to it so that neither nurse nor patient can leave, nor anyone enter without her knowledge.

All nurses should rank and be paid alike with progressive increases of wages after ten years' good service, or a slow annual increase which is better.

The nurse's rooms should be supplied with plain, comfortable furniture. In the large hospitals the head nurse furnishes her own room or rooms which doubtless promoted her comfort and her care of the furniture, both desirable things, yet the tendency of many to accumulate decorations which take time to clean etc. is a drawback. I should be inclined to try a furnishing plan or at least have some scale as to the furniture allowed. A bed, arm chair and sofa, a chest of drawers, wash hand table or shelf, book case or shelves, a little table and a larger one, a couple of chairs a footstool and a cupboard with broad shelves are the utmost that can be required.

Subsidiary Notes

Contrary to popular belief, Miss Nightingale was always in favour of a proper pension fund for nurses, though, at this early stage, she was doubtful as to how it could be worked out. She later approved Henry Burdett's scheme for a National Pension Fund. What she did not approve was the idea of paying certain nurses an honorary pension or stipend in lieu of wages as was at one time proposed by the St Katherine's charity.

Pensions for Nurses

'Apart from raising the wages of good nurses after every ten years' service, I think it would well answer to establish a graduated scale of pensions for both head nurses and nurses beginning with a small pension after ten years' good service increasing every five years afterwards. Many women are quickly worn out in this life; it is equally undesirable to turn faithful, worn-out servants adrift without any provision or to retain them for duties for which they have become unfit. It is a question whether there should not be compulsory stoppage from wages in order to entitle them to a pension under conditions.'

Subsidiary Notes as to the Introduction
of Female Nursing into Military
Hospitals in Peace and War, 1858

On the Importance of Female Staff Living in Rooms off the Wards

'This facilitates the manager's task, preventing gossip and promotes efficiency of nurses. . . . A common day room is undesirable. It encourages dawdling and gossiping. Her time ought to be fully occupied by her ward work, her necessary sleep and exercise and what making and mending she has to do for herself, for which time should be given her so that it may not be done on the sly. . . . Shut up all communication between the Nurses' Home and the hospital except through the street.'

to William Rathbone, 20 June 1860

'This [St Thomas's] is the only hospital where night nurses have no regular meals; (1) one before going on duty, one before coming off (2). No one to see they keep regular hours of sleep and exercise (3). They have no classes. Nurses too young are put on night duty and have no supervision on or off duty. There should be one extra nurse to every surgical ward.'

to Henry Bonham Carter, 1875

'It is far more difficult to induce a "middle class" woman than an upper class one to go through as a Head Nurse, the incidental drudgery which must fall to the province of the Head Nurse or be neglected.'

to Dr William Farr, 1866

'No Lady Superintendent be she upper, middle or lower class is qualified to govern or train nurses if she herself has not gone through the training of a nurse.'

ibid.

On the Importance of Ward Sisters as Teachers of Probationers

'I think we must consider seriously
  1. Whether we should not make a decided stand to have our probationers *only under Sisters* who are deliberately *approved* on wards essential to our training.'

to Henry Bonham Carter, 1873
(The Fund paid all sisters who had
probationers on their wards an extra
£10 a year whether or not they had any
ability for teaching or not.)

'It is all very well to put the Lady Probationers to exactly the same work as the others Viz, housemaids work.

I W'd not relieve them of emptying slops & the like, this is strictly Nurse's work. But the rest I would.

And in spite of the jealousies of the other pros Lady Ps must be relieved in the afternoon from 2–6 pm and be exempted from housemaid's work.

We intend the Lady Ps for a different course – we hold out to them a different future – from others And yet we give them no means by which to prepare themselves for it . . . '

Indeed they are so wearied that they fall asleep at Mr Croft's Classes at 8 pm.'

to Henry Bonham Carter, 1873
(The probationer's day was 7 am to
8.30pm with 2 hours off duty if work
permitted.)

In her dictum that the 'lady must train with her cook', Florence Nightingale was hoist with her own petard. The idea that the better educated should be specially groomed for 'superintendence' never materialised because of hospital jealousies and rivalry and the fact that they were valuable as biddable labour on the wards. This is a dilemma that Florence Nightingale did not solve, nor did her successors until the RCN initiated a Ward Sister's Course after the introduction of the National Health Service, and even then comparatively were able to benefit from it. The question of a two tier recruitment by educational standards continued to cause controversy and recrimination in the profession for the next hundred years.

11

Last Words

Although Florence Nightingale was thought to be at death's door when she was 37 years old, she lived to the age of 90 years. Until she was almost in her late fifties she described herself as 'an incurable invalid' with what she called 'The Thorn in the Flesh'. In spite of what Sir George Pickering [1] and Professor Barry Smith [2] have said it seems that she continued to have episodes of nausea, palpitations, insomnia, neuralgia and severe spinal pain and there were days when she could not work or see anyone. Another aspect of her illness was irritability and depression, although whether this was *post hoc* or *propter hoc*, it is difficult to say. Then round about the age of 60 years she seems to have undergone a metamorphosis. The thin, waspish woman given to acrimonious and tart retorts blossomed into a stout and benevolent old lady.

In 1875, after the death of her father, she left South Street to sort out the family affairs, complaining that it took her away from her work, and, at the same time became her mother's champion. Relations with Parthe had improved and she was a frequent visitor to Claydon and the Verney family, and she showed an interest in what was going on at the Nightingale School. However, she never cast off her invalid regime, she continued to see only one person at a time and then only by appointment, and although it was now possible to contradict her, one suspects that a visit to Miss Nightingale was like approaching the Delphic oracle.

Why did this change come over her? It was not, as has been suggested, because the family strains and conflicts had ceased. Parthe had been safely married since 1858 and letters show that generally her relationships with her parents had been affectionate for some time. Nor, as far as we know, was her treatment any different, though it may have been more positive. Was she, as has been suggested, a burnt-out case of brucellosis? Or was the change hormone related? We will never know. What does seem likely, however, is that her restless and often irritable personality after 1857 was at least in part related to her 'Crimean Fever'.

Until she was in her late seventies, Miss Nightingale kept up a lively interest in India, the Army politics, metaphysics and nursing. In some things she remained remarkably forward looking; in others she was stubbornly reactionary. She never accepted the germ theory, the need for women's suffrage or the idea of examinations for nurses. Her attitude to the young was a mixture of indulgence and censoriousness. (Witness her exhortations to young nurses in 'The Addresses'.) She was, however, an indulgent aunt and much loved by her younger nieces and nephews, even though they played hockey.

As far as St Thomas's was concerned, once Miss Pringle had left and joined the Church of Rome and had resigned as matron in 1889, her interest began to wane.

The new matron was chosen without consulting her, and both she and the Fund were being sidelined. However, she kept up a correspondence with a number of old Nightingale nurses like Florence Lees, Mary Crossland and Rachel Williams, though, on the whole, what she heard about nurses she did not like.

Unfortunately this benign state was soon to be clouded by failing memory and eyesight. By the time she was 80 years old she could only read and write with difficulty. Soon there would be no more words of wisdom or dogmatic assertions, and for the last years of her life she was confined to her bedroom in South Street overlooking the park, which she could not see.

One thing she was adamant about was that those who came after should learn the lessons of the past and look to the future. The last thing she wanted was to be the 'Nightingale Tradition', or indeed, to be a portrait on the back of a ten-pound note [1].

'Resignation, I have never understood the word.'

Private note, 1847

'I had previously refused all solicitations to give them 'relics' of me and the Crimean War on the grounds that the relics were:

1. *Sidney Herbert's*, R Commission & 4 Sub-Commissions which laid the imperishable seed of the great improvements in the soldier's daily life – direct & indirect.
2. the training of nurses both in character and technical knowledge. The untrained nurses sent out to the Crimean War were – well, it is unspeakable what they were.
3. the Hygiene & Sanitation the want of which in the Medical & Military author-ities caused Lord Raglan's death & that of thousands of our men from disease.'

to Edmund Verney, 1897

'*She* felt it a privilege, not a sacrifice, to attend the sick. Every Nurse must do so. Or she is not worth her salt . . .

'It is a great truth that we love those we make happy whether loveable or not.'

to Julia Ann Elizabeth Roundell, 1896
(On the subject of a 'Life of Agnes
Jones'. This is an example for how Miss
Nightingale changed in her old age. At
the time of Agnes Jones's death she was
sarcastic about 'the fussy maundering
accounts' and that 'her [Agnes's] mind
was going some months before her
death'.)

'I do not wish to be remembered when I am gone.'

to Henry Bonham Carter, 1859
(On the subject of the statuette.)

'Tell [Charles] Kingsley that the Protestant doctrine that to be disappointed in love or in search of love is a qualification for a good nurse or sister is nonsense; these women make infamous nurses.'

to Mr Nightingale, 1862

'The War office deserves the V.C. for cool intrepidity in the face of facts.'

Comment on the passing of the
Contagious Diseases Act 1864

'Oh happiness like Bread Fruit Tree, what a corrupter of human nature you are.'

to May Mohl, 1867
(On observing Lord Stanley now mar-
ried, happy, complacent and obese – an
excuse for a tirade against marriage.)

'We were perfectly right to begin as we have done to have our aim defined . . . the reform of hospital nursing was essential as a beginning. . . . But I would never look upon the reform of hospital nurses as an end rather only a beginning.'

to Henry Bonham Carter, 1867
(Referring to community nursing)

'I have a superstition as far as myself am concerned "against images made by hands". I would rather leave no memorial of my name or anything else.'

1868
(On refusing a request for a
photograph.)

'(Col: 6) As *every*body ought to have a defined "Occupation", I wish to return mine.

I ought, at least, to put "War Hospital Matron or Hospital Matron retired from active service thro' illness" (?)

I asked a Government friend what I should return. And he said that, the object being to classify industrial occupations, I ought to return "None Gentlewoman".

In all three assertions I am quite sure he is wrong . . . M. Mohl used to call me: "Empress of Scavengers for India and the British Kingdom".

If I were to put Scavengeress for India & the United Kingdom it would be near the truth. But – *what shall I do? what shall I return?'*

to Sir Harry Verney, 31 March 1871
(On the Census Form.)

'I must remember that God is not my Private Secretary.'

Private note, 1874, and repeated later

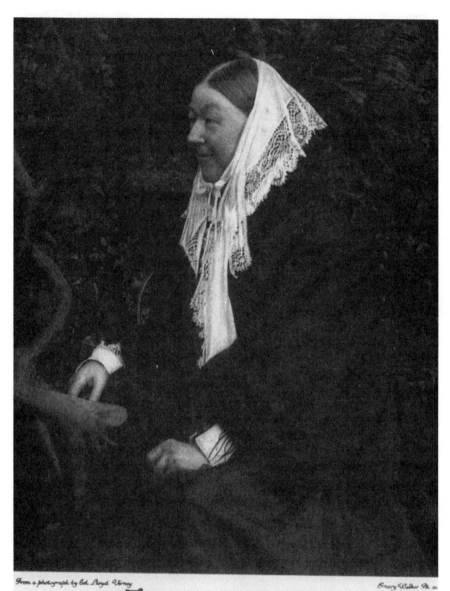

From a photograph by Col. Lloyd Verney   Emery Walker Ph. sc.

Florence Nightingale.

A photograph of Florence Nightingale taken at some time during the last decade of her life by Colonel George Lloyd-Verney and reproduced by photogravure in 1911 for purchase by readers of the *Nursing Times*.

'While Sanitary measures give perfect immunity from Smallpox, Vaccination does not . . .

Vaccination tho' it does not protect from Smallpox as Sanitary measures do, appears to protect in a measure from *Death* by smallpox. . . .

The anti-Vaccinators' liberty of-the-subject cry against compulsory Vacc'n is absurd. I only wish there were more that was *compulsory* – such as house-to-house visitation of sinks etc. etc. . . .

(I like Garibaldi cannot pass the Ho. of C. without tears) & we pray for all those who are working for a Ho. of C. that shall serve Him.'

to Sir Harry Verney, 18 March 1880

'We are not sent, are we? except to the lost sheep of the house of – Britain.

Is it not a higher "enterprise" to be District Nurse to "25" poor Holborn "families" than to "25 agricultural families" in E. Africa or even to be a trained Sister in a Hospital Ward?'

to Angelique Pringle ('the Pearl'),
1 March 1888
(This is apropos of Miss Formby
wanting to do a course of midwifery in
order to look after twenty-five families in
East Africa. While Miss Nightingale was
'enthusiastic about Emigration' (she
wrote much on the subject), she was
convinced that it should be to give the
poor or 'women on the verge of
Prostitution' a new start – our 'lost
sheep'. Emigration should not take away
the able and the best labourers.)

'Let me remember that as Mrs Nield is to me so I am to God.'

Private note, 1889
(Mrs Nield was Miss Nightingale's
excellent cook.)

'I have raised your wages to £15 (per annum) tho' I had cause, as you know to suffer from your want of skill. I hope to raise them to £16. And if I find when I come home that you have put something in the Savings Bank and that you have done well in your now somewhat responsible post I hope to be able to add to your nest-egg in the Sav'gs Bank.'

to Frances Groundsell, 1884
(Miss Nightingale believed in training
her servants in thrift. In this case young
Frances, like Oliver Twist, asked for
more, only to be the recipient of a long

and reproachful letter, ending with
'One would have thought that, merely
out of self-interest, you would have
known better than to write such a
letter'.)

'A flannel stomach belt I think a great protection.'

to Miss Munro, 1888
(Giving advice on suitable clothing for
the Egyptian campaign.)

'Is not Socrates ineffably tiresome?'

to Benjamin Jowett, 1889
(On the Georgias.)

'Shall I royally disregard it – or send them a Buster?'

Henry Bonham Carter, 1890
(On a letter berating her for opposing
registration.)

'I do not know what to do but ask you . . . '

to Henry Bonham Carter, 1890
(A frequent opening when Miss
Nightingale did not know what to do or
was contemplating doing something
rash.)

'You have never been Mother-in-chief to St Thomas's. You take the Cross and you use it as a club to give blows. . . . I have *never* been Thy Servant, I always seek my own glory – not thine.'

Private note, January 1890
(When depressed about nursing.)

'No gentlewoman ever wears anything but real lace.'

to one of Shore Nightingale's daughters,
1892

'Nursing has become a fashion, an amusement, a talk, or a literature – a dress.

E.g. at the recent Oxford meeting with the Pr. [Princess Christian Helena] as President some ladies were quite shocked at the Nurses – noisy, untidy, exclaiming "worth while to belong to the R.B.N.A. for the pretty badge" & this tone pervading everything. There was not one they said, like a Nurse of the (not modern) Schools. This is grevious – the public will take them for the crème de la crème – & they are not even skim milk.'

> *to Frances Spencer, Superintendent*
> *Edinburgh Royal Infirmary, 16 August*
> *1893*

On Nurses

'There is a *fashion* now in Nursing. . . . The *modern* tendency seems to be to let nurses out like Plumbers – for so many hours a day on the wards . . . & then let them live for the remaining hours quite apart from the hospital. . . .

[There is also] the tendency to substitute the literary nurse for the practical nurse. . . . then there is the giving lectures *first & last* – which is putting the cart before the horse or teaching Greek before English.'

> *to Frances Spencer (who had become*
> *Lady Supt in Edinburgh) 1893*
> *(This is a reference to Mrs Strong's*
> *Preliminary Training School started at*
> *Glasgow Infirmary, of which Miss*
> *Nightingale disapproved.)*

'It is perhaps but little known that in more than one London Poor Law Infirmaries long years after her death (Agnes Jones) there was a throwing of tin cups and plates across the ward by the Patients at each other, then giving the other in charge to the police.

All this disappears when there are educated women as Matrons & Ward Nurses. All really trained women are educated women.

But another danger appears now: the Doctors say: 'those women know as many words as we do – but they don't know how to make a patient comfortable.'

> *to Julia Ann Roundell, 1896*
> *(Having come round to the view that*
> *nurses must be educated, Miss*
> *Nightingale, like many after her, feared*
> *that knowledge and theory would be at*
> *the expense of practical skill and*
> *dedication.)*

'Nurses are quack nurses.'

> *Note, 1895*
> *(On some district nurses.)*

'The probationers are all loud and nasty. They have no holiday in the first year and one day off a month.'

> *to Mary Crossland (retired), 1896*
> *(On the current regime at St Thomas's*
> *of which she disapproved.)*

'He [Lord Shaftesbury] would have been in a lunatic asylum if he had not devoted himself to reforming asylums.'

to Margaret Verney, 1896

'111. Revision of the Old & New Testaments – I like to hear of it. It has always seemed to me that some of the alterations in the *New* are unpardonable, e.g. in the Lord's Prayer "But deliver us from *evil*" is altered to the "evil one". We always want to shift everything on to the devil . . . '

to Edmund Verney, 10 March 1897

'The "relics" and "representations" of the Crimean War! What are they? They are, first, the tremendous lessons we have had to learn from its tremendous blunders and ignorances. And next they are trained nurses and the progress of Hygiene. These are all "representations" of the Crimean War. And I will not give my foolish portrait (which I have not got) or anything else as "relics" of the Crimea. It is too ridiculous. . . . I won't be a sign at an Exhibition. Think of Sidney Herbert's splendid Royal Commissions which struck the keynote of success in the British Army! Think of the unwearied toil of the Sanitarians. . . . And you ask me for a photograph of a rat! And at the moment when there is Plague in Bombay!'

On being asked for pictures and relics
for the Victoria Era Exhibition, 1897
(The portrait by Barrett now hangs in
the National Portrait Gallery and
appears on the £10 note.)

'How inefficient I was in the Crimea! Yet He has raised up Trained Nursing from it.'

Private note, 1898
(On the Exhibition as being an occasion
for giving thanks to God.)

'He was a most interesting man, but you could never teach him sanitation.'

Private note, 1898
(On an interview with the Aga Khan.)

'I never did anything except when asked.'

to a young friend, [?] 1900

'As for riding, no hockey, no games will equal it for improving the circulation . . . So drat hockey and long live the horse. Them's my sentiments.'

to Margaret Verney, 1900

'No memorial whatever should mark the place where lies my Mortal Coil and my body should be given for dissection on post mortem examination for the purposes of Medical Science.'

Last Wish, [?] *1904*

Too kind, too kind.'

to the King's representative on receiving
the Order of Merit, 1907

References

[1] Pickering Sir G (1974) *The Creative Malady*. London: Allen & Unwin.
[2] Smith F B (1982) *Florence Nightingale – Reputation and Power*. London: Croom Helm.

Who's Who
among some of Miss Nightingale's correspondents

Acland, Henry, M.D. (Sir) 1815–1900

Regius Professor of Medicine at Oxford, who published widely on sanitation and medical education. He was involved in medical politics and the subject of registration. Miss Nightingale corresponded with him often, particularly on the subject of midwifery.

Bonham Carter, Henry, 1827–1921

The third son of John and Joanna Bonham Carter (Fanny Nightingale's sister) and the brother of the beloved Hilary. He was educated abroad and at Trinity College, Cambridge. He was a Unitarian and read law, being called to the Bar in 1853. He became Managing Director of the Guardian Life and Fire Assurance Company. This enabled him to give time to the Nightingale Fund, which he served as secretary from 1861 to 1914, retiring at the age of 87. He had eleven sons and one daughter, many of whom had distinguished careers. It is Henry's regular correspondence with Miss Nightingale that supplies us with our best source material on the Nightingale Schools. Henry himself became an authority on nursing and was largely responsible for the smooth running of the school and calming the oft-troubled waters at St Thomas's. Henry showed great prescience in understanding the independent role of the nurse.

Bracebridge, Selina, 1800–1874

Miss Nightingale met Selina Bracebridge in 1846, through Clarkey (Madame Mohl, *q.v.*). The Nightingale family encouraged the association, with its literary and social connections. Selina was happily married to Charles Holte Bracebridge, and both were indefatigable travellers and upholders of liberty; Charles had taken part in the revolt of the Greeks against the Turks. Miss Nightingale accompanied the Bracebridges to Rome and later to Egypt and Greece, and they arranged her visit to Kaiserswerth. Later, they came out to Scutari to help 'living in pigging conditions'. Miss Nightingale always said that Selina was more than a mother to her. Charles was a trustee and Council member of the Nightingale Fund, and both he and Selina visited the school and sent back reports to Miss Nightingale. Charles had warned about giving the matron, Mrs Wardroper, too much power, and was in favour of a more independent and professional training scheme.

Bowman, Professor Sir William, 1816–1892

The most distinguished ophthalmic surgeon of his day and an anatomist, giving his name to the capsule that surrounds the renal glomerulus. He was appointed to the staff of King's College Hospital in 1840, and was partly instrumental in the foundation of St John's House institution for nurses. He met Miss Nightingale at Harley Street when she assisted him with a difficult operation. He tried to persuade her to come to King's College as the superintendent, which she might have done had she not gone to the Crimea. William Bowman was an original member of the Nightingale Council and served it diligently. He was partly responsible for the Fund's Midwifery School at King's College, and, in spite of the School's unhappy end and the controversy, he and Miss Nightingale remained on close, friendly terms. Dr Bowman made a number of visits to the Nightingale School at St Thomas's. He was knighted in 1883.

Bunsen, Christian Carl Josias von, 1791–1860

An immensely wealthy Prussian theologian, diplomat and scholar of ancient and oriental languages who applied his philological knowledge to the study of the scriptures. In 1817 he entered the diplomatic service in Rome under the Prussian Ambassador, the historian, Barhold Niebuhr, where he met Thomas Arnold, Richard Monckton Milnes and a number of English intellectuals who were later to contradict the Church's teaching on the chronology of the scriptures. In 1842 he became Ambassador to the Court of St James where, through her parents, he met Florence Nightingale, with whom he and his wife, Frances, became close friends. It was Bunsen who suggested that she study nursing at Kaiserswerth. Bunsen played an important role in the religious discussions of the time. He introduced Max Müller to Oxford, who, with his *Sacred Books of the East* did much to widen the religious views of educated men. Bunsen was in attendance at the case of George Cornelius Gorham, who like Maurice, had questioned baptismal regeneration. Gorham's appeal that his views were not contrary to the Church were upheld, a decision to which Florence Nightingale makes reference in *Suggestions for Thought*. It was the decision that finally caused Henry Manning to embrace the Church of Rome.

Canning, Lady Charlotte, 1817–1861

Together with Lady Laura Cranworth and Elizabeth Herbert, she was responsible for the interviewing and hiring of the nurses for the Crimea. She was on the governing body of the Harley Street Institute, and Florence Nightingale kept up a long correspondence with her about her ideas on nursing management and the running of the establishment. She married Earl Canning, a Peelite Tory, who became the First Viceroy of India.

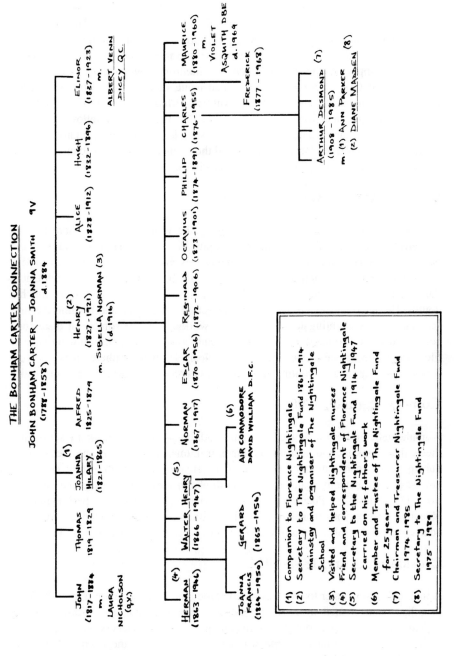

THE BONHAM CARTER CONNECTION

JOHN BONHAM CARTER = JOANNA SMITH qv
(1788-1858)   d.1884

JOHN (1817-1884) m. LAURA NICHOLSON (qv)

THOMAS 1819-1829

JOANNA HILARY (1) (1821-1865)

ALFRED 1825-1879

HENRY (2) (1827-1721) m. SIBELLA NORMAN (3) (d.1916)

ALICE (1828-1912)

HUGH (1832-1896)

ELINOR (1827-1923) m. ALBERT VENN DICEY QC.

HERMAN (4) (1863-1946)

WALTER HENRY (5) (1866-1947)

NORMAN (1867-1917)

EDGAR (1870-1956)

REGINALD (1872-1906)

OCTAVIUS (1873-1901)

PHILLIP (1874-1891)

CHARLES (1876-1955)

MAURICE (1880-1960) m. VIOLET ASQUITH DBE d.1969

FREDERICK (1877-1968)

JOANNA FRANCIS (1864-1956)

GERARD (1865-1956)

AIR COMMODORE DAVID WILLIAM D.F.C. (6)

ARTHUR DESMOND (7) (1908-1985) m. (1) ANN PARKER (2) DIANE MADDEN (8)

(1) Companion to Florence Nightingale
(2) Secretary to The Nightingale Fund 1861-1914 mainstay and organiser of The Nightingale School
(3) Visited and helped Nightingale nurses
(4) Friend and correspondent of Florence Nightingale
(5) Secretary to the Nightingale Fund 1914-1947 carried on his father's work
(6) Member and Trustee of The Nightingale Fund for 25 years
(7) Chairman and Treasurer Nightingale Fund 1974-1985
(8) Secretary to The Nightingale Fund 1975-1989

Chadwick, Edwin, 1800–1890 (K 1889)

A protégé of the Utilitarian philosopher Jeremy Bentham, and the secretary of the Poor Law Commission, and partly responsible for its philosophy. He became an ardent sanitarian, seeing a strong link between preventable ill health, pauperism and poor housing. With immense energy, he visited the worst slum towns and compiled statistics to support his theory. His report, *The Sanitary Conditions of the Labouring Population of Great Britain* (1842), remains one of the most informative Blue Books of the nineteenth century, and was known to Miss Nightingale. Chadwick was contumacious and an *enfant terrible* to the establishment, but as a fellow sanitarian, Miss Nightingale appreciated him and corresponded with him on many matters, including the Poor Law. They both regarded the germ theory with suspicion, fearing it would undermine the belief in sanitary principles.

Clough, Arthur Hugh, 1819–1861

An outstanding pupil of Dr Arnold at Rugby, he went to Balliol, where he lost his religious faith and threw up his fellowship. His uneasiness increased with the practice of poetry, and he became the principal of University Hall, London. In 1854, he married Blanche, daughter of Aunt Mai (Mrs Samuel Smith, *q.v.*) and Uncle Sam, and became attached to Miss Nightingale, who seemed to understand his doubts. He made himself useful to her, correcting her proofs, and became the first secretary of the Nightingale Fund Council, working out the somewhat disastrous contract with St Thomas's when he was already a sick man. The following year in Florence, at the age of 42, he died of tuberculosis. He is remembered for some fine lyrics. Miss Nightingale continued to take an interest in his family until her death.

Comte, Auguste, 1798–1857

A mathematician born in France who, in 1830, in *Cours de Philosophie* set forth a thesis that mankind had seen three stages in human thought: (1) the theological, during which mankind seeks to explain the supernatural by inventing gods and devils; (2) the metaphysical, in which he thinks in terms of philosophical abstractions; (3) the last, The Positive or scientific, when he proceeds by experimental and objective observations to reach a positive truth. Positivism attracted a number of adherents and disciples, but as the century moved on they became fewer in number.

Crossland, Mary, 1837–1914

Appointed Home Sister to the Nightingale Home in 1875; she retired in 1895. This post had been created in 1872 as Matron's Assistant, but Mrs Wardroper had resisted this, and three people had come and gone in quick succession. It was left to Miss Crossland, a former governess, to carve out a role for the Home Sister. This involved conflict with Mrs Wardroper, and Miss Crossland was a frequent visitor to

South Street and a regular correspondent, who kept Miss Nightingale informed about what was happening in the school and of her worries about the welfare and progress – or lack of it – of the probationers. The correspondence continued after Miss Crossland retired.

Farr, Dr William, 1807–1891

A pioneer in the new science of medical statistics and a member of the Army Health Board, Miss Nightingale enlisted his help to make comparisons of the sickness and death rates in barracks with those in civilian life. Dr Farr was an important member of the Barrack Commission, and worked closely with Miss Nightingale on the Royal Sanitary Commission on the Health of the Army in India. Dr Farr recognised that Miss Nightingale alone had the facts that could bring about reform, and he became a close friend. He supplied her with many of the statistics for *Notes on Hospitals*, and they corresponded on many matters, including nursing.

Galton, Captain Sir Douglas, 1822–1899

A brilliant engineer with the Royal Engineers, a leading expert on barrack construction and a member of the talented Galton family. In 1851, he married the beautiful Marianne Nicholson, the cousin for whom Miss Nightingale once had a 'Passion'. Miss Nightingale recognised Galton's talent, and in 1862 persuaded the War Office to secure his appointment as Assistant Under-Secretary (with Galton resigning his commission) and to be in charge of the health and sanitation of the Army. This position, it was hoped, would enable him to carry on with some of Sidney Herbert's reforms. Miss Nightingale continued to correspond with Galton on sanitary matters, and often sought his advice on hospital construction. She took a life-long interest in the Galton family.

Herbert, Sidney, 1810–1861

The younger brother of the Earl of Pembroke of Wilton House, a staunch High Churchman, and much concerned with the welfare of his estates. In 1846 he married Elizabeth à Court, who shared his interests. The Herberts were friends of the Bracebridges, and they all met in Rome in 1847. Sidney Herbert was impressed with Miss Nightingale's knowledge of hospitals, and this led to visits to Wilton, where she became very friendly with Mrs Herbert. Sidney Herbert became Secretary of State at War in the Aberdeen administration, and thus bore the brunt of the criticism of the Crimean War. In 1854, at his wife's instigation, he was responsible for sending Miss Nightingale with a party of nurses to Scutari. In 1855 he became secretary to the Nightingale Fund appeal, and was the mainspring behind its organisation. After the war, he was made Secretary of State for War, and was in a position to effect some reforms in the Army. Because of his rapidly failing health, he gave up his House of Commons work, being created Lord Herbert of Lea in 1860. He continued to work for the Fund, and died at Wilton on 2 August 1861. His son, the Earl of Pembroke, became a member of the Fund Council.

Jowett, Benjamin, 1817–1893

Educated at St Paul's School and Balliol College, Oxford, he became Regius Professor of Greek in 1855 and Master of Balliol in 1870. In 1871 he published a translation of Plato, with which Miss Nightingale helped him. Miss Nightingale first made his acquaintance in 1860, when Arthur Clough sent him her *Suggestions for Thought* to read. Although *Suggestions for Thought* was a failure, it brought about a lasting friendship, and Jowett became an adviser who often curbed Miss Nightingale's more exaggerated flights of fancy and hyperbole. He was devoted to her, though there is probably no truth in the story that he asked her to marry him. Jowett used to administer the Sacrament to her in South Street, where she was sometimes joined by her family, and he became a visitor to Embley. Jowett, like Miss Nightingale, was a legend in his own day.

Manning, Henry Edward, 1808–1892 (Cardinal, 1875)

Educated at Balliol College, Oxford, and a Fellow of Merton. After years of doubt about 'the Anglican predicament', he joined the Church of Rome in 1851 and became Archdeacon of Westminster. He was an eminent preacher, and Miss Nightingale first met him in Rome in 1848 when she herself, for a short time, was attracted to the Roman Catholic Church as a way of fulfilling her 'missions'.

Martineau, Harriet, 1802–1876

The daughter of a Norwich manufacturer, a Unitarian, who began her literary career as a writer on religious subjects, but made her name writing stories to popularise economic subjects and social reform. She was an active journalist, contributing to the *Daily News* and the *Edinburgh Review*. Physically unattractive, deaf and without a sense of smell, she had great prestige and could count among her friends the main literary and political figures of the day. Like Miss Nightingale, she suffered from ill health, and, thinking she had an incurable disease, took to her bed for five years and was cured by mesmerism (hypnotism). Later, in 1855, she was said to be suffering from heart disease and retired to Cumbria, but lived for another twenty years. Miss Nightingale used her to further her reforms, although she did not always agree with her views on women's rights and forbade her to use *Notes on Nursing* as 'a sermon on pioneer women'. Unlike Miss Nightingale, who also went through various vicissitudes in religious belief, Miss Martineau became an agnostic.

Maurice, Frederick Dennison, 1805–1872

A friend of Bunsen and an important influence in the nineteenth century Church. In the light of the controversy surrounding Darwin he published a series of articles in which he declared that the search for truth was all important and was not incompatible with God's goodness. In 1853, because of his involvement in the dispute over baptism he was dismissed from his post as Professor of Theology at King's College; his sister Mary was on the Board at the Harley Street Institute and a friend of Florence Nightingale who threatened to leave the Church of England in protest. It was through Mary that she first met Maurice, whose views were much in tune with her own. In 1861 Maurice was involved with the cause célèbre over the case of Bishop Colenso of Natal who had expressed 'Lax views on Biblical inspiration' and had withdrawn his belief in eternal punishment, claiming he was following the teaching of Maurice, but Maurice's views were more thoughtful and subtle. Later Maurice became a founder member of the Christian Socialists, an attempt by religion to meet the problems raised for working men and to demonstrate that political activity did not lie outside the province of the Church. As a Professor of Moral Philosophy at Queen's College he had an important influence in the education of women and that important group of women social workers, including Beatrice Webb, towards the end of the century. Dennison Maurice was the prototype for Shaw's delightful Reverend Morell in *Candida*.

McNeill, Sir John, 1797–1883

Acquired considerable knowledge of the East when working as a medical officer in the East India Company. In 1855 he was sent with Colonel Tulloch to enquire into the management of the Commissariat in the Crimea, where he met Miss Nightingale. The report confirmed the allegations of mismanagement, but at home the Chelsea Board was set up to whitewash the criticisms. Miss Nightingale helped to swell the public indignation, and Sir John became her friend for life; he helped her with her evidence to the Army Sanitary Commission. Sir John was an original member of the Nightingale Fund Council and urged caution about the contract with St Thomas's. He retired to Scotland but remained a father figure to Miss Nightingale, and she corresponded with him regularly.

Mill, John Stuart, 1806–1873

The son of the philosopher, James Mill, who, like his father, became a writer on political economy. He started as a supporter of Bentham's Utilitarianism, but departed from that philosophy and veered towards socialism. He was a great supporter of the rights of women and published *The Subjection of Women* in 1869. He was the Rector of St Andrew's University, Scotland, and Liberal MP for Westminster from 1865 to 1868 when he retired to France. Like Miss Nightingale, who corresponded with him, he thought the Poor Law system 'rotten to the core'.

Although she did not agree with him on his stand on the rights of women, she sent him drafts of her writings for his comment.

Milnes, Richard Monckton, 1809–1885 (created Lord Houghton in 1863)

Educated at Trinity College Cambridge, where he was a friend of Tennyson, Hallam and Thackeray, he travelled widely and, like Miss Nightingale, was a great supporter of the Italian and Greek wars of independence. He entered Parliament in 1838, but wanted to write poetry, and, although he produced several volumes, his claim to fame is as the champion of others, particularly of Keats. He became a friend of the Nightingale family, and wanted to marry Florence, but she refused him. (He married the Hon. Annabelle Crewe in 1851.) He remained an admirer of Florence's talents, and was a most valued trustee of the Nightingale Fund. Easy going and affable with infinite good humour, he espoused a number of causes, the chief of which was the Boys' Reformatories, and he was also a trustee of the British Museum, but in spite of his many activities, he gave attention to the Nightingale School and visited it. His son, the Earl of Crewe, became a trustee in 1899.

Mohl, Julius von, 1800–1876

An aristocratic German and the leading orientalist of his day who translated the oriental classics into a European language for the first time. While staying in Paris he fell in love with the witty, intellectual Mary Clarke and became a French citizen to be near her. Eventually he supplanted Claude Fauriel and married Mary in 1847 (see 'Mohl, Madame'). Julius, like Mary, adopted the Nightingale family. Like Bunsen (*q.v.*), he helped with Florence's studies of other religions and he followed her career with interest until his death.

Mohl, Madame (Mary Clarke), 1796–1883

A figure in the literary and political world of Paris. 'Her great charm lay in her absence of it'; she was a friend of Madame Recamier, the celebrated wit and beauty of the French Restoration period (1820s). For a time, Mary lived *à deux* with the well-known scholar Fauriel. Meeting the Nightingales on a visit to Paris, she was attracted to the family, and particularly to Florence, and they remained firm friends. In 1847, 'Clarkey' married Julius Mohl (*q.v.*), an Oriental scholar, who also liked Florence and corresponded with her. Clarkey used her influence with Fanny Nightingale to gain Florence's freedom. She continued as a correspondent and confidante to the end of her life, and was the recipient of some of Miss Nightingale's more acerbic outpourings.

Moore, Mother Clare, 1814–1874

Joined the Mercy Institute in Dublin shortly after its foundation by Catherine McAuley in 1831 and worked with the Sisters coping with the cholera epidemic that ravaged Dublin in 1832. A Protestant by birth, Clare Moore was probably the most intellectual of the Sisters. In 1839 she moved to Bermondsey, one of the most deprived areas in London and, showing a talent for dealing with difficult personality problems, became the Superior. It was to her that Bishop Grant, the Bishop of Southwark, turned in response to the appeal in *The Times* for nurses for the Crimea. Mother Clare and four nuns left on 27 October on the understanding that they would be under the administration of Florence Nightingale appointed by the Secretary of State. Generally known as 'Mother Bermondsey', Mother Clare worked indefatigably throughout the war and was Florence Nightingale's greatest support; her nursing experience was invaluable and she in many ways was Miss Nightingale's teacher. The two women became close friends, both were interested in mysticism and kept up an exchange of books and letters on the subject until Mother Clare's death.

Nightingale, Frances (Fanny), 1778–1880

One of the ten children of William Smith, who sat in the House of Commons 'fighting for unpopular causes'. Smith was a leading Abolitionist, and counted William Wilberforce, the anti-slavery campaigner, among his friends. Fanny inherited his liberal tendencies and the 'passion for clever friends'. On marriage, Fanny hoped to be a political hostess to a circle of reforming and avant-garde friends, and in this she was largely successful. Florence may have despised her mother's way of life, but it was through her mother's social circle that she was able to count on the help of so many influential people in later life. Fanny was generous and warm-hearted, and, contrary to myth, was interested in Florence's activities, as her letters testify. Florence never hesitated to use her mother's generosity for her lame ducks.

Nightingale, Parthenope (Lady Verney), 1819–1890

Neither as pretty nor as witty as her sister, she did not shine in society in the same way. Nevertheless Clarkey (Madame Mohl, *q.v.*) was attracted to her, and described her as elegant. Once out of the shadow of her sister, she blossomed. She was helpful and intelligent about the Nightingale Fund, as her letters to Sidney Herbert show. Florence recognised that her sister had artistic talents that were undeveloped. When she became Lady Verney, she took a real interest in the family estate at Claydon, wrote the memoirs of the Verney family during the Civil War, five novels and some essays on agriculture, and produced some sketches which are worth seeing. Until she was crippled with arthritis, the two sisters corresponded more, and were closer, than biographers allow.

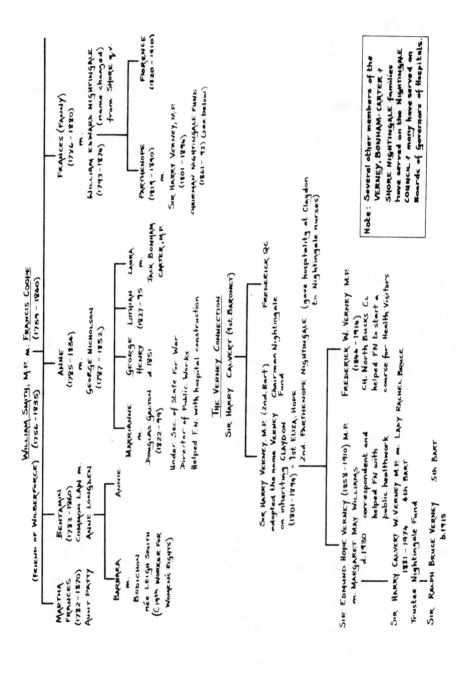

WILLIAM SMITH, M.P. m. FRANCIS COOPE
(FRIEND OF WILBERFORCE) (1756-1835)   (1759-1840)

MARTHA FRANCES (1782-1870)
Aunt Patty

BENJAMIN (1783-1860)
COMMON LAW m. ANNE LONGDEN

ANNIE

BARBARA m. BODICHON
née LEIGH SMITH
(19th worker for Women's Rights)

ANNE (1785-1824)
m. GEORGE NICHOLSON (1787-1852)

MARIANNE m. DOUGLAS GALTON (1822-99)
Under Sec. of State for War
Director of Public Works
Helped F.N. with hospital construction

GEORGE HENRY d.1851

LOTHIAN (1827-75)

LAURA m. JACK BONHAM CARTER, M.P.

FRANCES (FANNY) (1792-1880)
m. WILLIAM EDWARD NIGHTINGALE (1793-1874)
(name changed from SHORE q.v.)

PARTHENOPE (1819-1890)
m. SIR HARRY VERNEY, M.P. (1801-1894)
CHAIRMAN NIGHTINGALE FUND (1861-72) (see below)

FLORENCE (1820-1910)

THE VERNEY CONNECTION
SIR HARRY CALVERT (1st BARONET)

SIR HARRY VERNEY, M.P. (2nd Bart) adopted the name VERNEY on inheriting CLAYDON (1801-1894) = 1st ELIZA. HOPE
2nd. PARTHENOPE NIGHTINGALE

FREDERICK QC
Chairman Nightingale Fund

(gave hospitality at Claydon to Nightingale nurses)

SIR EDMUND HOPE VERNEY (1858-1910) M.P.
m. MARGARET MAY WILLIAMS d.1130
correspondent and helped FN with public healthwork

SIR HARRY CALVERT W. VERNEY M.P. m. LADY RACHEL BRUCE
1881-1974   4th BART
Trustee Nightingale Fund

SIR RALPH BRUCE VERNEY   5th BART
b.1915

FREDERICK W. VERNEY M.P. (1846-1914)
CH. North Bucks Co.
helped FN to start a course for Health Visitors

Note: Several other members of the VERNEY, BONHAM-CARTER + SHORE NIGHTINGALE families have served on the NIGHTINGALE COUNCIL + many have served on Boards of Governors of Hospitals.

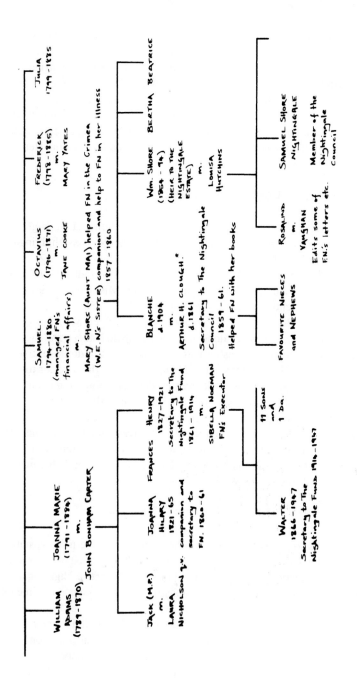

Two genealogical tables of the Nightingale family showing how Miss Nightingale's relations helped with her work. The list is not exhaustive; many other relatives helped with the Nightingale Nurses, and other relatives served on the Fund Council.

Nightingale, William (W.E.N.), 1794–1874

Miss Nightingale's father's original name was Shore, but he changed it to Nightingale on inheriting a fortune from an uncle of that name. He went up to Cambridge, which apparently transformed him, and in 1818 he married Fanny Smith, a great beauty, against the wishes of her family. W.E.N. was a cultivated man and interested in politics – he had stood for Parliament without success and he supported his neighbour, Lord Palmerston. He took charge of his daughters' education himself, for which Florence often thanked him. Miss Nightingale corresponded with her father on political matters, and she obviously valued his opinion. Her letters often show real affection.

Pringle, Angelique Lucille, 1842–1921

From a Scottish family, she came to train as a Special Probationer at the Nightingale School and proved to have outstanding qualities which caused Miss Nightingale to call her 'the Pearl'. In 1871 Miss Nightingale wrote 'I am afraid the only good sister (at S T H) is Pringle. Should we make her Wardroper's Assistant?' In 1872 Miss Pringle was sent to the Edinburgh Royal Infirmary as Miss Barclay's assistant to start a Nightingale School there. Following Miss Barclay's breakdown from addiction to opium and alcohol, and resignation a year later [1], Miss Pringle took over as Lady Superintendent. Almost alone of the Nightingale leaders, she succeeded in maintaining a harmonious relationship with the medical and administrative staff and produced a School of Nursing that Miss Nightingale thought superior to that at St Thomas's. In 1887 Miss Pringle took over as the Lady Superintendent at the Nightingale School at St Thomas's, but after a spiritual struggle she decided to join the Church of Rome and gave in her resignation much to the disappointment of Miss Nightingale and Jowett (*q.v.*) who had an agonising correspondence over her. Miss Pringle continued to correspond with Miss Nightingale and the letters form part of the Nightingale collection. Of all the 'Nightingales' Miss Pringle probably made the most significant contribution to nursing.

Quetelet, Lambert Adolphe Jaques, 1796–1874

A Belgian natural scientist who is regarded as the founder of modern social statistics and who organised the Commission Central de Statistique which led to the founding of the International Statistical Congress in 1853 of which Florence Nightingale was a member. His articles on 'social physics' demonstrated that age-specific crime rates were regular and can be discovered by statistics and these regularities have causes in social conditions in different places, this casts doubt on 'free will and the responsibility for crime'. Quetelet argued that legislation to improve social conditions would lower the crime rate. Florence Nightingale was attracted to this theory because she believed in the wholeness of the individual. Her passion for collecting statistics in the Crimea formed the basis of her report to the Royal Sanitary Commission.

Rathbone, William, 1819–1902

The eldest son in a dynasty of wealthy Liverpool shipowners. Unitarian by conviction, he retained his connection with the Quakers. He first approached Miss Nightingale in 1860, when he asked her advice about setting up a district nursing scheme. Three years later, he offered to finance a scheme for trained nursing at the Brownlow Hill Workhouse Infirmary. In 1868, William Rathbone became a Liberal MP and, now in London for part of the year, was largely responsible for promoting the Metropolitan and National Nursing Association. In 1877 he became a trustee of the Nightingale Fund, and took over the chairmanship on the death of Sir Harry Verney. Like Sir Harry, he played an active role, on Miss Nightingale's behalf, in the debate on registration. Together with Miss Nightingale, he was largely responsible for ensuring that the Queen Victoria Jubilee Institute, when it was established in 1887, promoted trained and professional district nurses under the control of a trained nurse superintendent.

Smith, Mrs Samuel (Aunt Mai), 1798–1889

Mr Nightingale's younger sister Mary, who married Fanny's younger brother, Samuel. In 1827, Aunt Mai gave birth to a son, Shore, who became heir to the Nightingale estates, and whom Miss Nightingale called 'my boy Shore'. Aunt Mai helped to persuade the family to let Florence study mathematics, and Florence became devoted to her. In 1855 she joined Florence in Scutari and helped her with the overwhelming clerical duties. When Florence was ill in 1857, Aunt Mai took her to Malvern and returned with her to London to 'look after her in her last months'. Eventually, after two years, and on the insistence of Uncle Sam, Aunt Mai returned home. Florence refused to speak to her and did not forgive her for twenty years. Nevertheless, Florence remained much attached to Shore and his family.

Stanley, Arthur Penrhyn, 1815–1881

Son of the Bishop of Norwich, he was educated at Rugby under the celebrated Dr Arnold, and then at Balliol College, Oxford. He became well known as the Dean of Westminster. His sister Mary went out to the Crimea with the party of ladies that was to give Miss Nightingale so much trouble. Dean Stanley asked Miss Nightingale to use her influence to dissuade Mary from joining the Church of Rome. Dean Stanley and his wife Augusta, who was a friend of Queen Victoria, were very interested in nursing matters and were involved with the setting up of the Queen Victoria Jubilee Nursing Institute.

Sutherland, Dr John, 1808–1891

A member of the McNeill Sanitary Commission in the Crimea and an authority on public health. When Lord Panmure tried to suppress the report, Miss Nightingale fought tooth and nail, and John Sutherland became her devoted ally. He was an important member of the Barrack Commission, and subsequently counsellor and medical adviser to Miss Nightingale. As her amanuensis, he came up from Norwood to sit in a downstairs room at South Street, often communicating with her by cryptic notes. Dr Sutherland often advised her on sanitary matters, helped to edit her books and travelled abroad on commissions. Although his deafness sometimes irritated Miss Nightingale, she relied on him and usually took his advice.

Verney, Frederick W., 1846–1913

Sir Harry's son by his former marriage, he became the chairman of the North Bucks. County Council under the new Local Government Act. It was through him that Miss Nightingale organised the first course for health visitors in a technical college. She became very attached to him and his family.

Verney, Sir Harry, 1801–1894

Elected MP for Buckingham in 1832, a seat he held almost continuously for 52 years. In 1858, he married Parthe Nightingale, Florence's sister, his first wife having died. As a Liberal and a reformer, he was interested in Miss Nightingale's work and became chairman of the Nightingale Fund Council. He remained in the post until 1890. He was assiduous in the Fund's affairs, and one of the highlights of the School's year was a visit to Claydon. In her later years, Miss Nightingale herself spent much time at Claydon and became attached to the various members of the family. There are about 4,000 Nightingale papers at Claydon, which is now National Trust property.

Verney, Margaret (Lady Verney), 1844–1930

The wife of Sir Edmund Verney, Sir Harry's eldest son, with whom Miss Nightingale became intimate, calling her 'The Blessed Margaret'. Margaret was not only beautiful; she was also a capable administrator, and it was through her that Miss Nightingale took an interest in the Claydon estate. There are a large number of letters addressed to Margaret.

Reference

[1] Baly M E (1986) *Florence Nightingale and the Nursing Legacy*. London: Croom Helm/Routledge.

Select Bibliography

Primary Sources

Held at the London Record Office (GLRO):
The Nightingale Collection. (Nightingale Training School).
The Nightingale Fund Council Records.
The records of St Thomas's Hospital.

Held at the British Library:
The Nightingale Collection.
The Rathbone papers.

Held at Wilton House:
The Herbert papers (vols 1855–61).

Held at Claydon:
The Verney Nightingale papers.

At the Wellcome Institute:
Selection of extracts from Nightingale letters on microfiche.

Writings by Miss Nightingale

Letters Written by Florence Nightingale in Rome in the Winter of 1847–48, Keele
  M (ed.). American Philosophical Society, 1981.
*Subsidiary Notes as to the Introduction of Female Nursing into Military Hospitals
  in War and Peace*. London: Harrison and Sons, 1858.
Notes on Nursing: What it is and What it is not, 2nd edn. London: Harrison and
  Sons, 1860.
*Suggestions for Thought to the Searchers after Truth among the Artizans of
  England*, 3 vols. London: Eyre and Spottiswoode, 1860 (privately printed).
Notes on Hospitals, 3rd edn. London: Longmans Green and Co., 1863.
*Suggestions on the Subject of Providing Training and Organising Nurses for the
  Sick Poor in Workhouse Infirmaries*. Report of the Committee on the Cubic
  Space of Metropolitan Workhouses, 1867.
'Una and the Lion', *Good Words*, June 1868.
*Introductory Notes on Lying-In Hospitals together with a proposal for the Training
  of Midwives and Midwifery Nurses*. London: Longmans Green and Co., 1871.

Addresses to the Probationer Nurses in the Nightingale Fund School at St Thomas's Hospital, 1872–1900, selection printed for private circulation.

On Trained Nursing for the Sick Poor. Spottiswoode and Co., 1881.

'History of District Nursing'. *A History of Nursing in the Homes of the Poor.* Introduction by Florence Nightingale in a book by William Rathbone, dedicated to Her Majesty on the foundation of the Queen Victoria Jubilee Institute. London: Macmillan, 1890.

'Nurses, training of and Nursing the Sick'. In Quain R (ed.) A *Dictionary of Medicine.* London: Longmans Green and Co, 1882, reissued 1910.

Books

Abel-Smith B (1960) *A History of the Nursing Profession.* London: WM Heinemann.

Baly M E (1995) *Nursing and Social Change*, 3rd edn. London: Routledge.

Baly M E (1986) *Florence Nightingale and the Nursing Legacy.* London: Croom Helm/Routledge.

Berlin I (1956) *The Age of Enlightenment* (C18th Philosophers). New York: Mentor Books.

Bonham Carter H (1862) *Suggestions for Improving the Management of the Nursing Departments in Large Hospitals.* Blades.

Bonham Carter V (1960) *In a Liberal Tradition: A Social Biography.* London: Constable.

Boyd N (1982) *The Victorian Women who Changed their World.* London: Macmillan.

Calabria M D and Macrae J A *Selections & Commentaries: Suggestions for Thought by Florence Nightingale.* Philadelphia: University of Pennsylvania.

Chadwick O (1980) *The Victorian Church*, Part II. London: Adam & Charles Black.

Cook Sir E (1913) *The Life of Florence Nightingale*, 2 vols. London: Macmillan.

Cope Z (1958) *Florence Nightingale and the Doctors.* London: Museum.

Forester M (1985) *Significant Sisters.* London: Penguin.

Huxley E (1975) *Florence Nightingale.* London: Weidenfeld and Nicolson.

Jowett B (1860) *Essays and Reviews* (eds Abbott E. and Campbell, L.). London: John W Parker & Son.

Martineau H (1869) *The Positive Philosophy of Auguste Comte.* New York: Gowans.

O'Malley I B (1931) *Florence Nightingale 1820–1856.* London: Thornton Butterworth.

Osborne H and Godolphin S (1855) *Scutari and its Hospitals.* London: Dickinson & Brothers.

Paton H J (1972) *The Moral Law.* London: Hutchinson University Library.

van der Peet R (1995) *The Nightingale Model of Nursing.* Edinburgh: Campion Press.

Pickering Sir G (1974) *Creative Malady.* London: Allen and Unwin.

Plato (1955) *The Republic* (translated by Desmond Lee). pp. 427–347. London: Penguin Classics.

Reid Sir T W (1890) *The Life and Letters of Richard Monckton Milnes, Lord Houghton*. London: Cassell.

Ricks C (ed.) (1987) *The New Oxford Book of Victorian Verse*. Oxford: Oxford University Press.

Smith F B (1982) *Florence Nightingale – Reputation and Power*. London: Croom Helm.

Strachey L (1918) *Eminent Victorians*. London: Chatto & Windus.

Summers A (1988) *Angels and Citizens: British Women as Military Nurses 1854–1914*. London: Routledge & Kegan Paul.

Vicinus M and Nergaard B (1989) *Ever Yours, Florence Nightingale Selected Letters*. London: Virago.

Webb B (1946) *My Apprenticeship*. London: Penguin.

Woodham-Smith C (1950) *Florence Nightingale*. London: Constable.

Woolf V (1929) *A Room of One's Own*. London: Penguin.

Unpublished Thesis

Prince J E *Florence Nightingale's Reforms of Nursing 1860–1887*. University of London.

Index